Time for Health Education

Kaarina Määttä & Satu Uusiautti (eds.)

Time for Health Education

PETER LANG
EDITION

Bibliographic Information published by the Deutsche Nationalbibliothek
The Deutsche Nationalbibliothek lists this publication in the Deutsche Nationalbibliografie; detailed bibliographic data is available in the internet at http://dnb.d-nb.de.

Library of Congress Cataloging-in-Publication Data
Määttä, Kaarina.
  Time for health education / Kaarina Määttä, Uusiautti, Satu (eds.).
    pages cm.
  ISBN 978-3-631-64935-0
  1. Health education. 2. Health education–Finland. 3. School health services. 4. Health promotion. I. Uusiautti, Satu. II. Title.
  LB3405.M23 2014
  372.37–dc23

                                                          2014000371

Printed with financial support of the University of Lapland.

Cover illustration designed by Satu Uusiautti and Kaarina Määttä.
First published in Uusiautti, S., & Määttä, K. (2013).
How to promote the healthy development of
human resources in children and youngsters?
European Journal of Academic Research, 1(5), 212-221.

ISBN 978-3-631-64935-0 (Print)
E-ISBN 978-3-653-04028-9 (E-Book)
DOI 10.3726/978-3-653-04028-9
© Peter Lang GmbH
Internationaler Verlag der Wissenschaften
Frankfurt am Main 2014
All rights reserved.
PL Academic Research is an Imprint of Peter Lang GmbH.

Peter Lang – Frankfurt am Main · Bern · Bruxelles · New York ·
Oxford · Warszawa · Wien

www.peterlang.com

Forewords

Health and healthy life styles are something that we all would like to induce in our youth and children. Health education at school is one way of implementing health promotion. However, for all good intentions, the subject of health education makes a contradictory part of education: health education has been included in other school subjects, such as physical education, or themes of health education have been discussed from a cross-curricular point of view.

In today's world, issues of health do not just mean healthy life style but cover a much more profound part of human beings' lives: health education is expected to provide holistic information and increase understanding about the communal and environmental health issues along with individual choices and minding for fellow humans.

Time for Health Education covers health education, its history, and present and future challenges. It represents new ideas and hands-on solutions of health education and also analyses of health capital and health literacy among the youth and children.

In Finland, health education became an established school subject in basic education, vocational education, and general upper secondary education in 2001, and the history of the subject of health education has quite long roots in the Finnish education. The Finnish health education has been considered a trailblazer and therefore, we think that this would be a topic of great interest worldwide.

We have asked experts of education, all graduated from the University of Lapland, Finland, to contribute their viewpoints in this book. All articles included in the book are based on the authors' studies and gone through rigorous international review process.

Brief Look at the Offering of the Book

The chapters of the book are to provide versatile viewpoints to health education. In the Introductory chapter, the editors of the book, Prof. Kaarina Määttä and Adj. Prof. Satu Uusiautti review the versatile concepts of health promotion and education. The purpose is to introduce the hierarchy and relationship between the core concepts that will help the reader to understand the perspectives presented in the book and also the overall field of health education as a part of health promotion.

In Chapter 1, former minister of education of Finland, Dr. Maija Rask et al. have a glance at the history of health education in Finland starting from the 17th century's hygiene instruction all to way to the formation of the modern school subject of health education. Actually, health education became an established school subject during her term as a minister of education.

Chapter 2 covers important health-related concepts and their definitions: Dr. Outi Hyry-Honka et al. discuss the role of health capital in health promotion and Dr. Ari Kunnari et al. expand the discussion of human capital with a new concept of the experience-based capital of physical exercise. Dr. Maija Rask et al. introduce a new innovation, the fourth level of health literacy.

Chapter 3 includes select examples of health issues among children and youth. First, Dr. Marika Savukoski et al. introduce ex-anorectics' survival followed by M. A. Sanna Hoisko et al.'s study of ever-worrying phenomenon at school, bullying. Both articles have a fundamentally positive starting point as they focus on the survivors' perceptions and experiences.

The last chapter turns eyes on educators and their role in health promotion. Dr. Teija Koskela et al.'s article reveals what school teachers themselves think about practical pupil welfare work. The article introduces a typology of how pupil welfare work can be included at school. The final article of the book, written by Adj. Prof. Satu Uusiautti and Prof. Kaarina Määttä, discusses human resources compiling an illustration of the elements of positive development.

Take Care – and Be Well!

Time for Health Education is aimed for everyone interested in issues of health education at any education level. The especial target groups are students of education and health care; teachers and educators, and school health care nurses at various school levels; and educational, schooling, social, and health care administrative authorities.

The purpose is to support educators' and teachers' work by introducing new concepts, ideas, and practical solutions of health-related educational studies and practices.

As Nordic educators, we were inspired by a cloudberry when thinking about the prerequisites of healthy development. Health is like a cloudberry fruit—precious, beneficial, and well-balanced. And most importantly, through relevant knowledge and education, available for all. Caring educators can support and kindle the flame of the development of positive health skills, but not without established structures of health promotion and health education for all children and youth across the world.

We thank all the contributors for fruitful and inspiring collaboration and Coordinator Paula Niemelä for her help with the formatting of this book.

23 Jan 2014 at the University of Lapland, Finland

Kaarina Määttä and Satu Uusiautti

Table of Contents

Authors

Sanna Hoisko, MA, Finland

Outi Hyry-Honka, PhD, Rovaniemi University of Applied Sciences, Finland

Teija Koskela, PhD, University lecturer, University of Eastern Finland, Finland

Ari Kunnari, PhD, University lecturer, University of Lapland, Finland

Kaarina Määttä, PhD, Professor, Vice-rector, University of Lapland, Finland

Maija Rask, PhD, Kemi, Finland

Marika Savukoski, PhD, Director, Municipality of Keuruu, Finland

Satu Uusiautti, PhD, Adjunct Professor, University of Helsinki, Finland

Publication Details of the Articles

Määttä, K., & Uusiautti, S. (2013). The value and implementation of health education in Finland. *International Journal of Sciences, 2*(12), 46-51.

Rask, M., Uusiautti, S., & Määttä, K. (2013). Health – The first prerequisite of the joy of life. The history of the subject of health education in Finland. *History of Education & Children's Literature, 8*(3), 415-431.

Hyry-Honka, O., Määttä, K., & Uusiautti, S. (2012). The role of health capital in health promotion. *The International Journal of Health Promotion and Education, 50*(3), 125-134.

Kunnari, A., Määttä, K., & Uusiautti, S. (2013). Introducing the concept of the experience-based capital of physical exercise (ECPE). *Global Journal of Human Sciences, 13*(2), 15-23.

Rask, M., Uusiautti, S., & Määttä, K. (2014). The fourth level of health literacy. *International Quarterly of Community Health Education, 34*(1), 51-71. (Baywood Publishing Company, Amityville, New York)

Savukoski, M., Määttä, K., & Uusiautti, S. (2012). Back to life: How to use positive psychology to beat anorexia. *International Journal of Research Studies in Psychology, 1*(2), 39-51.

Hoisko, S., Uusiautti, S., & Määttä, K. (2012). How to overcome bullying at school? – The adult survivors' perspective. *International Journal of Academic Research in Business and Social Sciences, 2*(10), 58-72.

Koskela, T., Määttä, K., & Uusiautti, S. (2012). Pupil welfare work in Finnish schools – Communal or falling apart? *Early Child Development and Care, 183*(9), 1311-1323.

Uusiautti, S., & Määttä, K. (2013). How to promote the healthy development of human resources in children and youngsters? *European Journal of Academic Research, 1*(5), 212-221.

The Value and Implementation of Health Education

Kaarina Määttä and Satu Uusiautti

Health promotion is a global issue and different countries have implemented a wide range of health promotion campaigns. Concern over health behavior in youth, unhealthy life styles, and repetitively perceived problems in health have aroused discussion over how to support the youth in their pursuit for good life.[1,2,3]

The health behavior, health, and well-being in Finnish youth have been studied systematically already from the 1970s. In addition to separate national surveys[e.g.,4], numerous case studies on the youngsters' health skills[5,6] and school health surveys[e.g.,7] have provided plenty of information. Likewise, international studies of World Health Organization (WHO) have provided comparison information about the health behavior and well-being at school among the fifth-, seventh-, and ninth-graders since the 1980s[8,9]. The international European Network of Health Promoting Schools (ENHPS) program has evaluated the promotion of health of school communities, school health care nurses' health counseling and health education, and students' health learning both in Finland[10,11,12] and internationally[3,13,14].

The international discussion of the promotion of health education has been dominated by evaluations of various health programs and projects[e.g.,15,16]. Although schools aiming at health promotion were established in Europe (e.g., European Network of Health Promoting Schools, ENHPS)[17] and in the North-America (e.g., "Co-ordinated school health Programme")[see e.g. 18] already in the 1980s, they could not solve health problems in a way that was expected[19,20]. Although health definitions have been developed in many disciplines[e.g., 21,22] as well as means of measuring health[e.g., 23,24], still the connection between health skills in practice and in theory has proven problematic[25]. New research-based innovations are needed[26].

The realization of health education can be difficult also because of the amplitude of concepts and their overlap. The variety in terms can be explained by the multi-disciplinary nature of the phenomenon: health is studied in medicine, nursing, psychology, education, sport, sociology, and etcetera. Moreover, the practices of health education are quite differently emphasized in various countries.

The purpose of this article is to review the concepts of health education, analyze the connections between the concepts, and introduce the realization of health education in Finland. Finland is a pioneering country in health education because health education is a legally defined school subject in basic education (including elementary and secondary education), and in general and vocational upper secondary education. Health education is also included in the core curriculum of preschool education.

Viewpoints to the Amplitude of Concepts

Health education aims at health promotion. Health promotion can be seen as a wide main concept or an umbrella concept[24,27]. Then, the school subject of health education is one of the forms of implementing health education, and health education one of the strategies of promoting health[28,29].

We have illustrated the entity of health education through the various concepts and their mutual hierarchy (see Figure 1). As the following chapters will show, there are numerous concepts that could be included in the figure but we have carefully chosen the ones we find the most important to illustrate the connection between health promotion, health education, and eventually, the individual person's health skills. Health skills include health awareness, health sensitivity and health literacy. The fundamental idea is that at its most concrete, successful health promotion leads to high-level health skills that are manifested as the ability to cherish health and well-being at the level of the behavior of individual people and communities. At the individual level, health skills are symbolized with the flame of life as the outcome of health promotion, health education, and the school subject of health education. Next, we will define the current terms and introduce Finnish solutions to strengthen health education.

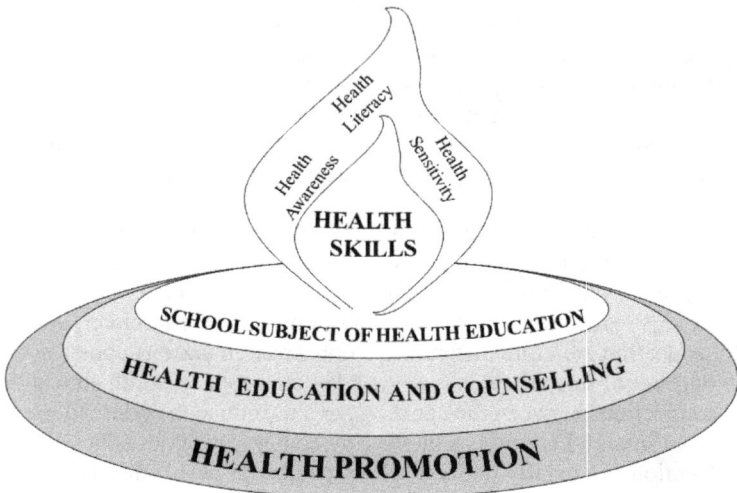

Figure 1. Core concepts of health education

Health Promotion

Health promotion is a multidimensional concept covering at least (1) health promoting and enabling measures and (2) preventive measures that are to prevent the development of illnesses, treat, and rehabilitate[e.g., 22,30]. The goal of the first is to strengthen the outer and inner factors that nurture health[e.g., 31]. The goal of health promotion is embedded in the health culture[e.g., 32] and written in health policies[e.g., 33]. Actually, today's public health and health promotion researchers are calling for better training and a stronger research culture in health policy as well[34]. This is because health promotion is under constant development internationally and interpreted by countries quite variedly.

Indeed, Signal states that "health promotion is an inherently political enterprise"[33, p. 257]. Health promotion is based on the declarations and programs of WHO world conferences[e.g., 35,36,37]. In Finland, the Council of State made a decision in principle in 2001 about the "Health 2015" national health program and the Ministry of Social Affairs and Health has compiled quality recommendations for health promotion in 2006. They aim at the promotion of the whole population, prevention of illnesses, and decrease of differences in health among population groups.

Health Education and Counselling

One of the areas of health promotion is health education which means health promotion through education, teaching, and informing[e.g., 24]. The purpose of it is to guarantee people with sufficient knowledge about the promotion and maintenance of good health and increase their interest in and skills of making decisions concerning their health. Health education wants to mold health behavior and attitudes in the population the goal being the adaptation of healthy life styles[38]. The ultimate purpose is to secure children's healthy and risk-free development and growth and lay the foundation for good health and well-being in adulthood. In practice, this means health appreciation and respect for the cherishing of health and for people with different health conditions through conversations about values, appreciations, and ideals[28,39].

In Finland, health education became an independent university-level subject at the University of Jyväskylä in 1990. Since the school year of 2006, Master-level education in health education has, in addition to other students of health profession, accompanied five students aiming at teachers of health education. Health education is concretized with the school subject of health education that has become a part of Finnish basic education.

Health Education as a School Subject

As mentioned, health education became an established school subject in Finland in 2001 Education[40]. The history of health education is long in Finland[41]. The current Finnish national core curriculum is a pioneering one among the solutions of implementing health education in school[41]. Other countries where local education is guided by national core curricula are England, Scotland, New Zealand, Singapore, South-Africa, and Sweden[42]. Still, the emphases and the ways the content is integrated in other subjects seem to vary between these countries. The United States, Australia, and Canada have no nation-wide curricula but state-specific curricula[42], and health education is often tied with health promotion programs in schools in the United States[43] and in Canada[44]. Likewise, giant steps in health education have been taken in China[45] and in Bangladesh[46]. In Finland, health education is divided into the actual health education and health promotion, the development of social skills and general life-management skills, and safety education[41,47]. In addition, health is an important content of preschool education[48].

The goals and contents of the school subject of health education are written in the National Core Curriculum for Basic Education[40]. According to the curriculum, the purpose of health education is to advance awareness that supports health, well-being, and security. Therefore, it also aims at developing cognitive emotional regulation, and functional and ethical readiness. To do that, the core contents of health education are (1) growth and development (life span; physical, mental, and social health; special features of adolescence development; and care for one's own health), (2) healthy choices in everyday situations (nutrition; smoking, alcohol, and other drugs; sexual health; human relationships; infectious diseases, illnesses; road safety; accidents and first aid), (3) resources and coping skills (health; work and work ability; emotions and expression of emotions; social support; interaction skills; crises of development and life phases), and (4) health, society, and culture (national diseases; environment and health; well-being at work; basic health care and welfare services; civic organizations; legislation about children's and youngsters' rights and limitations). Instruction of health education is based on the understanding of physical, mental, and social capability[40].

The teacher of health education is required to possess considerable knowledge and expertise. Kannas[29] defines those areas of health education that also determine the professional knowledge and expertise required but health education teacher: (1) visionary knowledge according to which the teacher has to have a clear vision and understanding of the core concepts and their interconnectedness of health education, health promotion, and health awareness; (2) lifestyle knowledge according to which the teacher should get the youth to adopt sensible, healthy habits; (3) methods knowledge according to which the teacher has to have suitable pedagogical skills including diverse teaching, communication, education, and guiding skills required of a health education professional; (4) strategic knowledge according to which the teacher has to have a holistic perception of the measures with which schools can promote pupils' and school personnel's health; 5) cultural knowledge according to which the teacher has to able to view critically phenomena related to health and illnesses also from the societal perspective; and (6) knowledge of health and illnesses according to which the teacher has to know what causes and what prevents diseases, and what are the most common diseases. The teacher of health education therefore works also as a health educator[29].

Caring teacherhood that supports well-being in pupils is important in health education, too[49,50,51,52,53,54]. Moreover, a health education teacher set an example!

In all, health education is a special school subject because of its experiential and emotional sensitivity. Topics discussed in lessons can be very personal, touching, and emotional. Therefore, a health education teacher cannot just rely on his or her knowledge of health issues and development of substance knowledge. At the same time, the teacher has to pay attention to challenges and needs related to pupils' age and developmental level.

In a school community, every teacher and student has their own values that direct their choices. However, the school shares common basic values to which teachers and students commit according to the curriculum. In Finland, the National Core Curriculum defines the teaching and education goals and the basic values for schools.

Health Skills

We use the concept of health skills to cover the elements of health awareness, health literacy, and sensitivity and other related concepts that each contribute an important part of an individual person's capability to cherish his or her health. As the illustration of Figure 1 implies, health education provides people with health skills that are manifested as high-level health literacy[55,56], health awareness and sensitivity even leading to empowerment[57,58]. Empowerment enables participation, active action, and becoming heard both at the individual and communal levels[59,60]. The individual people's responsibility over healthy choices increases, readiness to set personal health-related goals becomes strengthened, and experiences of coping skills, capabilities, and perceived social support increase[30]. Health education provides information about topical health risks and their avoidance and can prevent national diseases in adulthood. Therefore, health education can have significant economic influence in the form of citizens' ability to work and function[29,61].

Discussion: Challenges of Health Education

In order to sufficiently guarantee each and every individual person's health skills and decrease differences in people's health behavior and attitudes, the position of health education and health education teachers should be strengthened at school. Teachers need readiness to encounter diverse pupils and skills for supporting their well-being at social, emotional, and physical level. All these should be paid more attention to already during teacher training. Caring teacherhood[50,51,52,53] and sincere wish to strengthen pupils' positive resources, provide experiences of success, and boost pupils' trust in their skills and importance of their choices might be even more important than mastery of the contents of the school subject of health education[see also 61]. On the other hand, teachers' in-service training can be especially fruitful when it comes to the increasing knowledge of health education[26]. Health educators are required to have special professionalism and competence that is strengthened both along with their training and work experience[62].

Teaching methods should be developed to activate pupils and having them taking the responsibility over their own health behavior[see 27]. Dialogues with pupils[63,64,65] and focus group discussions[66,67] have proven successful methods of health education – within all the busy school life, these methods would deserve conscious effort and invest both in teacher training and at basic school. Especially, boys' health skills and their promotion necessitate special attention: according to research, they do not seem very interested in cherishing their health [19,41,68]. This concern over men's health has already given birth to a special journal to discuss the topic, namely the American Journal of Men's Health[e.g., 69].

The ethos of schooling should transmit the accepting and caring atmosphere that would be manifested through positive interaction and cooperation[70] and health-promoting leadership[71,72]. School should have special rewards for well-being promoting actions and measures. Along with various active and goal-oriented collaborative activities, the school personnel and pupils would cherish and strengthen health, well-being, and satisfaction at school[see 15].

It is also necessary to bring the knowledge acquired by research in health sciences into the practice of education[73] and show how significant health awareness for the quality of life and well-being is. Widening health literacy[19], appreciation of capital of physical exercise (see Chapter 4) and understanding health education as a part of health capital (see Chapter 3) make specific contributions to health promotion. Likewise teachers' and students' experiences of critical health threats make way to the discovery of successful solutions to change the progression in a positive direction (see Chapters 6 and 7). The aforementioned viewpoints exemplify research conducted at the University of Lapland, Finland, aiming at fostering vivid and innovative research on health education and teaching.

Active developmental aspirations that are grounded on the idea of caring, love-based school can be used for creating healthier school, a healthier new generation, and healthier future – toward a world where it is safe to live, love and take care of each other.

References

1. Berntsson, L. T., & Köhler, L. (2001). Long-term illness and psychosomatic complaints in children aged 2-17 years in the five Nordic countries. Comparison between 1984 and 1996. *European Journal of Public Health, 11*(1), 35-42.
2. Lightfoot, J., & Bines, W. (2000). Working to keep school children healthy: the complementary roles of school staff and school nurses. *Journal of Public Health Medicine, 22*(19), 74-80.
3. Morberg, S., Dellve, L., Karlsson, B., & Lageström, M. (2006). Constructed space and legitimacy for health work in the educational system: Perspectives of school nurses. *International Journal of Qualitative Studies on Health and Well-being, 1,* 246-244.
4. Joronen K. (2005). *Adolescent's subjective well-being in their social contexts.* (PhD Diss., University of Tampere, Tampere, Finland.)
5. Hakala P., Rimpelä A., Salminen J., Virtanen S. & Rimpelä M. (2002). Back, neck and shoulder pain in Finnish adolescents: national cross sectional surveys. *British Medical Journal, 325*(5), 743–746.
6. Rimpelä, M., Ojajärvi, A., Luopa, P., & Kivimäki, H. (2005). *Kouluterveyskysely, kouluterveydenhuolto ja terveystieto* [Survey on well-being at school, school health care, and health education]. Helsinki: National Institute for Health and Welfare.
7. Lintonen T., Rimpelä M., Vikat A., & Rimpelä A. (2000). The effect of societal changes on drunkenness trends in early adolescence. *Health Education Research, 15*(3), 261–269.
8. Konu A., & Rimpelä, M. (2002). Well-being in schools - a conceptual model. *Health Promotion International, 17*(1), 79-87.
9. Välimaa R. (2000). *Nuorten koettu terveys kyselyaineistojen ja ryhmähaastattelujen valossa* [Perceived health in youth according to surveys and group interviews]. Jyväskylä: University of Jyväskylä.
10. Tossavainen, K., Turunen, H., Jakonen, S., Tupala, M., & Vertio, H. (2004). School nurses as health counselors in Finnish ENHPS Schools. *Health Education, 104*(1), 33-44.
11. Turunen, H., Tossavainen K., Jakonen S., Salomäki U., & Vertio H. (1999). Initial results from the European Network of Health promoting Schools program on development of health education in Finland. *Journal of School Health, 69*(10), 387–391.
12. Turunen, H., Tossavainen, K., Jakonen S., Vertio H., & Salomäki U. (2000). Improving health in the European Network of Health Promoting Schools in Finland. *Health Education, 100*(6), 252–260.
13. Van Driel, W. G., & Keijsers, J. F. (1997). An instrument for reviewing the effectiveness of health education and health promotion. *Patient Education and Counseling, 30*(1), 7-17.
14. Moon, A. (2002). Health promoting schools and healthy schools awards. *Promotion & Education, 9*(1), 25-28.
15. D'Onise, K., Lynch, J. W., Sawyer, M. G., & McDermott, R. A. (2010). Can preschool improve child health outcomes? A systematic review. *Social Science & Medicine, 70*(9), 1423-1440.

18

16. Hackbarth, D., & Gall, G. B. (2005). Evaluation of school-based health center programs and services: the whys and hows of demonstrating program effectiveness. *Nursing Clinics of North America, 40*(4), 711-723.
17. Ziglio, E., Hagard, S., & Griffiths, J. (2000). Health promotion development in Europe: Achievements and challenges. *Health Promotion International, 15*(2), 143-154.
18. Allensworth, D. (1997). Improving the health of youth through a coordinated school health programme. *Promotion & Education, I*, 42-47.
19. Rask, M., Määttä, K., & Uusiautti, S. (2013). The challenges of health education: how to cherish health according to Finnish students' perceptions? *Problems of Education in the 21st Century, 51*(51), 91-103.
20. St Leger, L. (2004). What's the place of schools in promoting health? Are we too optimistic? *Health Promotion International, 19*(4), 405-408.
21. Jamner, M. S., & Stokols, D. (2000). *Promoting human wellness: New frontiers for research, practice, and policy.* Los Angeles, CA: University of California Press.
22. Nordenfelt L., & Liss P.-E. (Eds.) (2003). *Dimensions of health and health promotion.* New York, NY: Rodopi.
23. Green, L. W., & Lewis, F. M. (1986). *Measurement and evaluation in health education and health promotion.* San Francisco, CA: Mayfield Pub.
24. Sharma, M., & Romans, J. A. (2012). *Theoretical foundations of health education and health promotion.* Canada: Jones & Bartlett Learning.
25. Basch, C. E. (1987). Focus group interview: An underutilized research technique for improving theory and practice in health education. *Health Education & Behaviour, 14*(4), 411-448.
26. Leone, J. E., & Maurer-Starks, S. (2007). Innovative teaching strategies in research methods for health professions. *Californian Journal of Health Promotion, 5*(3), 62-69.
27. Callahan, D. (2000). *Promoting healthy behavior: how much freedom? Whose responsibility?* Washington, D.C.: Georgetown University Press.
28. Kannas L. (2005). Terveystieto-oppiaineen olemusta etsimässä [Looking for the essence of subject of health education]. In L. Kannas & H. Tyrväinen (Eds.) *Virikkeitä terveystiedon opetukseen* [Stimuli to the instruction of health education] (pp. 9-18). Jyväskylä: University of Jyväskylä.
29. Kannas L. (2006). Terveystieto-oppiaineen pedagogisia lähtökohtia [Pedagogical premises of the subject of health education]. In H. Peltonen & L. Kannas (Eds.), *Terveystieto tutuksi – ensiapua terveystiedon opettamiseen* [Familiarize with health education – first aid to health education] (pp. 9-36). Helsinki: Hakapaino.
30. Laverack, G. (2004). *Health promotion practice, power & empowerment.* London: Sage.
31. O'Donnell, M. P. (1986). Definition of health promotion. *American Journal of Health Promotion, 1*, 4-5.
32. Pasick, R. J., D'Onofrio, C. N., & Otero-Sabogal, R. (1996). Similarities and differences across cultures: Questions to inform a third generation for health promotion research. *Health Education Quarterly, 23*(Suppl), S142-S161.
33. Signal, L. (1998). The politics of health promotion: insights from political theory. *Health Promotion International, 13*(3), 257-263.
34. Bernier, N. F., & Clavier, C. (2011). Public health policy research: making the case for a political science approach. *Health Promotion International, 26*(1), 109-116.
35. WHO. (1986). *Ottawa Charter for Health Promotion.* Retrieved from: http://www.who.int/hpr/NHP/docs(ottawa_charter_hp.pdf.

A Glance at the History of Health Education

Health - the First Prerequisite of the Joy of Life

Maija Rask, Satu Uusiautti and Kaarina Määttä

Health promotion aiming at preventing infectious diseases and promoting preventive health services has a long history[1]. In developing countries, health education directed toward these goals remains a fundamental tool in the promotion of health and prevention of disease while in developed countries, during the 1960s and 1970s, this early experience in health campaigning was directed toward promoting healthy lifestyles[2]. Whatever the fundamental target, education has been considered the necessary action to promote health and prevent diseases.

In Finland, health education became an established school subject in basic education, vocational education, and general upper secondary education in 2001. This development has had many interesting phases, which are studied in this article. In elementary education it was integrated in other subjects such as biology, geography, physics, and chemistry[3,4]. In the curriculum for general upper secondary education, health education is defined in the following manner:

> Health education is a school subject based on multidisciplinary knowledge and its purpose is to promote skills that support health, well-being, and safety. This knowledge in manifested as intellectual, social, functional, and ethical abilities and skills of emotional regulation and information acquisition. Health literacy includes the readiness to be responsible for the promotion of one's own and others' health. In health education of general upper secondary education, health and maladies and health promotion and illness prevention and treatment are considered from the points of view of the individual, family, community, and society.[3, p. 210]

The subject of health education is divided into the actual health education and health promotion, the development of social skills and general life-management skills, and safety education[5,6,7]. The purpose of health education is to get the young adopt healthy life style. The instruction is expected to further pupils' sensitivity toward health. It means health appreciation and respect for the cherishing of health and people with different health conditions. Therefore, it is also to promote tolerance, adaptation skills, ability to bounce back from losses and the ability to renounce are important themes in health education. Teaching involves conversations about values, appreciations, and ideals[8].

According to annual School Health Surveys, most of the Finnish students find health education interesting. For example, in 2009 School Health Survey, 75% of general upper secondary education students reported that health education had increased their preparedness to take care of health[9]. Likewise, international results show the importance of health research among children and the youth and information health and education professionals[10,11] and respectively information provided to the youth and its positive, health-related consequences[2].

But what is the history of the subject of health education? In this article, we review the history of health education in Finnish schools. The study leaned on archival and primary sources available at the Archive of Parliament of Finland and accessed via the Library of Parliament. The data were comprised of contemporary textbooks, decrees, circular letters, and curricula. Our purpose is to draw a historical picture of the development of the subject and to show the importance of the subject in general.

Roots Hark Back to the 17th Century

The first general upper secondary school of Finland, Collegium Aboense, was established in Turku in 1630. The school followed Bishop Isak Rothovious's curriculum called "methodus didactica", and it included teaching of botany and pharmacology[12]. The early secondary school legislation did not recognize health education as a subject. In 1649 Queen Christina gave orders concerning schooling and among them, physics education at general upper secondary schools had to include, along with logic, studies of human body and basics of health care. Still in the 18th century, the basics of anatomy formed a part of physics education[12].

In 1843, secondary schools were supposed to include several hours of gymnastics as a part of education. However, no references about actual health education could be found. In 1870s, gymnastic teachers' education was complemented with studies on anatomy and physics[13]. Of Finnish cities, Jyväskylä was the pioneer of health education[12]. Viktor Heikel was considered the father of physical education for he taught hygiene at the Jyväskylä coeducational school in the 1880s[14]. It is likely that the girls' school of Jyväskylä and the Finnish girls' school of Helsinki had hygiene education in the last years of the 1880s[13].

How was the Teaching of Health Education Reasoned at the Beginning of the 20th Century?

One of the advocates of health education was MD and Docent of School Hygiene Max Oker-Blom. He wrote the text book for school and home, *Outline of Health Education*. In his forewords, he mentions the following:

> Health education or hygiene has lately recognized as an important part of people's valuable knowledge. Indeed, health is so precious that everyone has a full reason to know the conditions of maintaining good health and the prerequisites and demands of its development.[15, p. ii]

Oker-Blom did not consider health just physical health but he gave directions of maintaining the hygiene of mental health as well. He noted that health "is the first prerequisite of the joy of life"[15, p. 7]. In 1912, he published an extended edition of the book he aimed to the masses. This book became the first textbook of hygiene at secondary schools, and the third edition of it in 1916 already following the methodical directions of the Finnish School Board. The book was a practical health care manual. Oker-Blom defined hygiene as follows: "Hygiene is a branch of medicine studying what promotes and what hinders or threatens health. Hygiene does not study illness and nursing but aims at nurtiring and promoting health."[15, p. 5] Oker-Blom complemented his production by publishing a 300-page-long *Hygiene* in 1916. The book was even regarded as a praiseworthy textbook of sex education[14].

At the beginning of the 20th century, knowledge about the anatomy and physique of a human being was considered important for the understanding of hygiene. Schools used German professor Otto Schmeil's 70-page-long book *Human being* for that purpose. It comprehensively introduced the skeleton, muscles, nervous system, senses, respiratory organs, blood and bloodstream, lymph and lymphatic system, digestion, and secretory organs. It did not have much health care advice and the few it provided were value-based. For example, Schmeil explains why problem drinkers suffer from stomach diseases and concludes: "Any thinking human being does not have to be reminded what results from these facts!"[16, p. 63] On the other hand, he provided a functional advice on eye care, valid still today: "Do not put too much strain on your eyes! Most of all, remember to have moments of rest at work every now and then and look far away which is necessary rest for your eyes."[16, p. 31]

In the 1910s Gymnastic Teachers acted as Pioneers

Officially, the hygiene and temperance education started in Finnish schools on the 1st of October 1913.The senate decreed health education at secondary schools in 1911, 1912, and 1913. The Finnish School Board specified decrees by its circular letters to secondary school rectors in 1912, 1913, and 1914.[13]

In the circular letter dated 16 Jan 1914 in Helsinki, contemporary gymnastic teachers were ordered to be nominated as junior lectors of hygiene and temperance education. The first gymnastic teachers had graduated after the three-year-long education in 1911. Gymnastic teachers, who had relatively wide knowledge about hygiene and remedial sciences, already that time demanded separate lessons of hygiene in schools[14]. In the fall 1913, hygiene and temperance education started in Finnish schools by replacing one fifth-graders' gymnastic lesson by one lesson of hygiene and temperance education in the sixth grade. Suomela wrote that when at the threshold of the First World War hygiene and temperance education was included in the state and private school curricula, temperance education was taken care of much better than in the 1950s, at the time Suomela wrote his study[14].

Iwar Wilskman was selected as the associate inspector of gymnastic and hygiene education in 1914. The position regularized in 1918. Wilksman regarded that hygiene education included too much anatomy and physique, and lacked an up-to-date textbook, too[13].

Looking for the Essence of Hygiene at the Turn of the 1910s and 1920s

The circular letter of the Finnish School Board in 1917 defined the requirements of hygiene and temperance education in the following manner: "Education introduces the most important issues of common health care in individuals and the society, and provides pupils with information that is easy to remember […]"[13, p. 11]

Ivar Wilskman wrote *Hygiene* to be used in schools. His book was published in 1919. In his beginning sentence, Wilskman notes that Oker-Blom's *Outline of Hygiene* has little information about anatomy and health care advice. Wilskman says he knows how to structure hygiene education and what the textbook should be like. He justified his arguments by his work at the Finnish School Board where he had listened to 169 teachers' hygiene lessons. Wilskman defined health education as hygiene[17]. According to his definition, it is a science that teaches us what we must know and notice if we want to nurture our health properly, have a long life, and fully enjoy our existence.

Wilskman described the structure of a human body at length. His health care advice was directions that included long lists and appreciations. For example, he had included 23 directions under the title of *How to take care of your nervous system*. The directions could go as follows: «perform determinedly and promptly all your tasks that are your duty although you might find them repellent» or «always try to be satisfied and take the phases of life lightly; calmly and patiently tolerate hardships». Wilskman also suggests that certain grades should have two hours of hygiene education per week[17].

Wilskman rewrote *Hygiene* together with Professor of medicine Arne Palmén. In this book, Palmén and Wilskman divided hygiene into individual hygiene that was concerned of maintaining the healh of individual people; general hygiene that covered societal means of fighting against health threats; and racial hygiene aiming at securing the health of future generations. All branches of hygiene were interconnected as, for example, one's disease can affect other members of the society and even the future generations[18]. Palmén and Wilskman also warned about excessive health ethusiasm over health:

Sometimes health is overly cared. A person who sees health threats everywhere and thinks about his or her health all the time is unhealthy as such. The best for a human being is to follow simple and moderate life habits, have varying exercise for all organs of his or her body and rest, and, without being too strict, cherish his or her physical and mental health.[18, p. 219]

Physiologist Robert Tigerstedt's text book *Hygiene Education for Secondary Schools* (1921) had, unlike the title implicates, very little health care advice. Hygiene was not defined in this book. The first twenty chapters discussed the structure of a human body, and the last chapter introduced infectious diseases and their prevention. The book ends in a chapter called *Death and Decomposition*: "The whole living nature forms a uniform entity and every creature as a part of it has its special task to perform."[19, p. 218]

The State Regulations at the End of the 1930s

The law on Finnish state secondary schools (218/1939, §8) states that secondary education includes among others gymnastic and sport, civil defense, and hygiene and temperance education. The 1941 decree determined learning goals and methodical directions for state secondary schools. The purpose of gymnastic, sport, and hygiene education was to

> let pupils understand the meaning of health and health care for an individual and the nation, raise them physically and mentally healthy, eligible for work and defense, harmonious and flexible, and habituate them with healthy life style and adopt healthy and teetotal habits.[13, p. 12]

School children's physical shape was improved in PE lessons but civil defense was also included in teaching. Moreover, education was supposed to ignite and deepen pupils' patriotism. This way, the national goals influenced the way teaching of various subjects was arranged.

In 1948, the Finnish School Board gave directions on hygiene education to secondary school rectors and for the information of private school administers. The letter talks about actual health education. Health care and its meaning, the overall structure of a human body, sport, and nutrition and digestion had to be taught to fourth-graders altogether 15 hours. Fifth-graders were supposed to have one lesson per week covering respiration, bloodstream, secretion, skin and clothing, endocrine, nervous system, senses, dwelling and stimulants, and in girls' schools, also child care and household work. The spring semester of the seventh grade had 20 hours of health education. It consisted of themes such as infectious and national diseases, the meaning of health and temperance to society, and advanced studies in the most important issues of health care. Whenever appropriate, secondary education had to discuss first aid and the prevention of accidents. In addition, the directions said that if the teacher of health education considers himself or herself familiar enough with the theme and pupils, he or she can introduce the questions of sex education and racial hygiene at a general level in the fifth grade and more profoundly in the seventh grade education (Circular Letter of the Finnish School Board 1948, no. 1736).

School Hygiene and Integrity

More often than not, authors of hygiene textbooks justified the publication of their own book by the lack of a proper text book. Kari and Suomela did the same in the first edition of *Textbook for Secondary School Hygiene Education* in 1933. The authors had deliberately included less anatomy and physiology to highlight practical health care. They also emphasized temperance education and tuberculosis. In the tenth edition of their textbook, the authors stated that the task of civilized society is to cure the ignorance of health and health care through teaching and instruction. In addition to individual, general, and racial hygiene, they mentioned school hygiene that covered school-related health care and a part of general hygiene[20]. The book followed carefully the 1948 circular letter of the Finnish School Board. With the exception of Schmeil's *Human being*, all aforementioned textbooks included nutrient charts.

The 1959 circular letter named courses in temperance education, first aid, home-based nursing, becoming a family member, and environmental hygiene. General health care covered issues such as household maintenance, waste management, food supply, water supply, national nutrition and national diseases, alcoholism and international health care operation[13].

The program of physical education for girls that was confirmed in 1967 did not have directions on health education while boys' physical education program was introduced in 1960–1961. Health education that was included in physical education aimed at providing pupils with understanding about the significance of healthy life style. They were to adopt such healthy habits as sufficient exercising, appropriate clothing, taking care of cleanliness and tidiness, paying attention to dining, work, recreating and rest, and behaving safely and politely at school, in sporting places, and in traffic. Especial focus was in integrity. Teachers of various subjects had to do their best to create a school environment that would promote physical and mental health[13].

Nutrition and Responsibility on Focus in the 1960s

In 1964, Annikki Karvonen and Martti J. Karvonen[21] wrote in the forewords of *Health Book for Elementary School* that their book will introduce health care questions more extensively than other textbooks by cutting the proportion of anatomy and physiology. Anatomical pictures reminded pupils of body organs that they have already learned in zoology. The pictures summoned up the information and left time for the study of health care issues.[21] This book covered first aid in case of accidents. In addition, it introduced nutrients and the actual healthy nutrition in the form of a food circle. However, it does not contain information about the suitable and healthy proportions of each food stuff. Illnesses were introduces as well; most attention were given to infectious diseases, rheumatoid arthritis, cancer, and parasites. Mental illnesses are only mentioned as the consequence of alcohol abuse[21].

Another textbook from the 1960s was *You and Your Health*. Authors Margareta Hannula and Kerttu Larjanko mention in their forewords that the purpose is not only to maintain and improve pupils' health but also to be responsible for others' health, too. The book dedicated one chapter to sex education. Illnesses are introduced respectively after each anatomical and physiological issue. The book also had a chapter about looks and the effects of going to sauna[22].

In 1965, Holger Hultin concluded that hygiene forms a part of health education[23]. Hygiene provides pupils with knowledge about the structure of human body, way human being's function, and what can disturb it. Moreover, health education gives the so-called life manual and skills of considering health issues when making decisions. Hultin also used concepts of integrated and correlated health education. Integrated health education discussed a certain topic within other or all school subjects. In correlated health education, a topic was already part of the actual subject but connected to health education.

Hultin and Lyyli Virtanen published *Hygiene for General Upper Secondary Education* in the beginning of the 1970s. The main headings of the book were *Becoming an Adult, Reproduction, Health and Illness*, and *Healthy Lifestyle*. What was new about the book were the extensive recommended literature lists at the end of each chapter. The authors thought that the book was not suitable to ordinary classroom teaching but merely it was to support self-study and possible classroom discussions based on students' questions and interests[24].

Integrating Health Education in Other School Subjects in the 1970s

The strong position of health education was broken in the 1960s and 1970s. Scientific studies started to doubt the influence of knowledge about threats on the attitudes and behavior of children and the youth. As the national core curriculum for comprehensive education in Finland was compiled, hygiene was no longer a separate school subject but it was integrated mostly in civic education. This solution did not turn out to be functional and time allocation for civic education was decreased[25].

The subject of civics was introduced in elementary education at the beginning of the 1970s and when the suggestion of cutting the teaching of the subject was introduced at the end of the 1970s, the subject was supposed to consist of health and safety education, and teaching of manners[25].

Health Education of the General Upper Secondary Education written by Juho Korhonen, Tuula Eloranta, and Esa Santala followed the 1981 core curriculum for general upper secondary education. The book differed from the previous textbooks because it had a comprehensive chapter of environmental health care[26]. In 1985, the core curriculum integrated health education with civics in elementary schools and with physical education in middle schools. It meant that civic education was no longer provided in middle schools[6,25].

The 1993 subject allocation for schools defined the goals of education as thematic entities, one of which was health education covering for example healthy lifestyle and sex education[6]. The 1994 national core curriculum did not have a subject-specific curriculum for civic education. Health education was integrated in the school subjects of biology, physical education, and home economics. In the 1990s, the responsibility over curricula was given from the state to municipalities which meant in practice that health education diminished while the number of other optional studies increased in schools[25].

The Turn of Millennia

As the school laws were renewed in 1998, the parliament of Finland added health education in the subjects of general and occupational upper secondary education. Konrad Reijo-Waara who worked actively for the strengthening of health education in the 1890s stated already then that having hygiene education at school is an inevitable requirement of modern times[27]. Hence, Reijo-Waara's demand came true after a hundred years when health education was introduced as an independent subject in Finnish comprehensive education, and general and occupational upper secondary education in 2001.

Health education has had many names along its history: mostly in Finland, it has been called hygiene (Circular Leeter of the Finnish School Board 1914; Circular Letter of the National Board of Education 1948). The subject was called hygiene and temperance education already in 1913[14]. Later on, in the 1970s, health education had the name of civics[25], until health education became a separate subject in the general upper secondary education in 2001. This study showed how the health education had different emphases depending on the contemporary emphases. In Finland, the shift ranged from the discovery of the subject in the 17th century through national educational purposes at times leaving only minimal room for health education. At other times, health education was connected to other themes: especially at the first half of the 20th century, patriotic spirit, national solidarity, and volition to defend one's country were cherished at school[28]. It was also closely connected to temperance education as the purpose was to make the nation healthier and produce good and sober workers: one way of transmitting the ideology of temperance among the people was, naturally, education[29]. Teachers were in central role as they could control and cultivate pupils' physical and mental health[30,31]. In addition, health education was a part of gymnastics and physical education. Naturally, the goals of enhancing individual and national health was in line with the purposes of physical education, too[32,33]. As the historical-contextual background, it is worth noticing that some common societal tendencies seemed to be springing up across the world around the end of 19th and the beginning of 20th century[34,35,36]. In Finland, health education was also included in civic education, too, as it covered also the themes of for example environmental health and general health.

At the present moment, health education is a subject of its own. The purpose of the subject is to strengthen the teaching of health education as a part of basic education and to reach the whole generation, and thus to have a positive influence on the national health. Today, health education is divided in three parts: actual health education and health promotion, development of social skills and general life skills, and achievement of safety skills[15].

Conclusion

The foundation of youngsters' health appreciation is laid at school[37]. Information, skills, and values provided at school and at home form a strong basis for individuals' life styles and ways of nurturing their health[7]. Health education and healthy life style can be taught within various school subjects, but in addition, school transmits students the prevailing health-related knowledge, skills, attitudes, and values[38,39,40,41]. The importance of the subject of health education is justified in various ways. Health literacy is a part of all-round education[42].

Within the fast changes of the modern society, children need strong basis for maintaining and promoting their overall well-being. Today's world sets a new spectrum of threats to people's health[43]. Adults have to cope with the insecurity and stress, burnout and lassitude caused by rapidly changing modern working life: at the same time, for example, increasing unemployment and other societal problems pose demanding challenges for people's well-being and health. Furthermore, not only among adults but also among children and youngsters a variety of problems occurs: depression, exclusion, psycho-social problems, mental problems, and especially the increase in learning difficulties are worrying[44]. According to Kickbusch[45], a significant part of the world's population, even in the richest countries, is still ill-equipped to deal with a rapidly changing society when it comes to their knowledge about health issues. While the positive connection of education and health is widely recognized, it is also relevant to see that health is a complex system requiring a wide range of knowledge and skills. The school has an important role and the subject of health education has an important place in education when considered from this point of view. How to develop the subject in the future, then? To be able to strengthen youngsters' resources and health capital with various actions, we have to know what factors are relevant especially from the point of view of the young: what is the level of health capital[46] or health literacy[2] of the youth?

References

1. McLeroy, K. R., Bibeau, D., Steckler, A., & Glanz, K. (1988). An ecological perspective on health promotion programs. *Health Education Quarterly, 15*(4), 351-377.
2. Nutbeam, D. (2000). Health literacy as a public health goal: a challenge for contemporary health education and communication strategies into the 21st century. *Health Promotion International, 15*(3), 259-267.
3. *The National Core Curriculum of General Upper Secondary Education.* (2003). Helsinki: National Board of Education.
4. *The National Core Curriculum of PreSchool Education.* (2010). Helsinki: National Board of Education.
5. Government Bill. (142/2000) Retrieved from FINLEX data base: http://www.finlex.fi/fi/esitykset/he/2000/20000142
6. Peltonen, H. (2005). Terveystieto-oppiaineen pedagogisia lähtökohtia [Pedagogical premises of the subject of health education]. In H. Peltonen & L. Kannas (Eds.), *Terveystieto tutuksi – ensiapua terveystiedon opettamiseen* [Familiarize with health education – first aid to health education] (pp. 37-52). Helsinki: Hakapaino.
7. Rask, M. (2012). *Lukiolaisten terveydenlukutaidon ja terveysarvostusten ilmeneminen* [The manifestation of general upper secondary education students' health literacy and health appreciation]. (PhD. Diss., University of Lapland, Rovaniemi, Finland.)
8. Kannas, L. (2005). Terveystieto-oppiaineen olemusta etsimässä [Looking for the essence of the subject of health education]. In L. Kannas & H. Tyrväinen (Eds.), *Virikkeitä terveystiedon opetukseen* [Stimuli to the instruction of health education] (pp. 9-18). Jyväskylä: University of Jyväskylä.
9. Aira, T., Kannas, L., & Peltonen H. (2008). Terveystieto [Health education]. In M. Rimpelä et al. (Eds.), *Hyvinvoinnin ja terveyden edistäminen lukiossa. Perusraportti lukiokyselystä vuonna 2008* [The promotion of well-being and health at general upper secondary education] (pp. 50-56). Helsinki: Edita.
10. Lowry, R., Wechsler, H., Galuska, D. A., Fulton, J. E., & Kann, L. (2002). Television viewing and its associations with overweight, sedentary lifestyle, and insufficient consumption of fruits and vegetables among US high school students: differences by race, ethnicity, and gender. *Journal of School Health, 72*(10), 413-421.
11. St Leger, L., & Nutbeam, D. (2000). Finding common ground between health and education agencies to improve school health: mapping goals, objectives, strategies, and inputs. *Journal of School Health, 70*, 45-50.
12. Malmio, B. (1933). *Luonnonopin opetuksen kehitys maamme oppikouluissa* [The development of natural science teaching in our secondary schools]. Helsinki: Otava.
13. Korhonen, J. (1971). *Katsaus terveyskasvatuksen kehitykseen Suomen kansa- ja oppikouluissa* [A look at the development of health education in Finnish elementary and secondary schools]. Jyväskylä: University of Jyväskylä.

14. Suomela, K. U. (1950). Katsaus terveysopin opetuksen vaiheisiin maassamme [Review of phases of hygiene education in our country]. *Kouluvoimistelu ja Urheilu, 1-2,* 7-9, 11-13.
15. Oker-Blom, M. (1910). *Terveysopin pääpiirteet. Oppikirja koulua ja kotia varten* [Outline of health education. A textbook for school and home]. Helsinki: Otava.
16. Schmeil, O. (1908). *Ihminen. Ihmisruumiin rakenteen ja terveysopin pääpiirteet* [Human being. The outline of the human body structure and hygiene]. (transl. W. M. Linnaniemi). Porvoo: WSOY.
17. Wilksman, W. (1919). *Terveysoppi kouluja varten* [Hygiene for schools]. Helsinki: Otava.
18. Palmén, A., & Wilskman, I. (1926). *Terveysoppi kouluja varten* [Hygiene for schools]. Helsinki: Otava.
19. Tigerstedt, R. (1921). *Terveysoppi: oppikouluja varten* [Hygiene education for secondary schools]. Porvoo: WSOY.
20. Kari, K., & Suomela, K. U. (1955). *Oppikoulun terveysoppi* [Textbook for secondary school hygiene education]. (10th ed.) Porvoo: WSOY.
21. Karvonen, A., & Karvonen, M. J. (1964). *Keskikoulun terveyskirja* [Health book for elementary school]. Porvoo: WSOY.
22. Hannula, M., & Larjanko, K. (1969). *Sinä ja terveytesi* [You and your health]. Helsinki: Otava.
23. Hultin, H. (1965). *Terveyskasvatus koulussa. Lapsi ja nuoriso* [Health education at school. Children and the youth]. Helsinki: Lastensuojelun Keskusliitto.
24. Hultin, H., & Virtanen, L. (1975). *Lukion terveysoppi* [Hygiene for general upper secondary education]. Helsinki: Yhteiskirjapaino Oy.
25. Rimpelä, M. (2000). *Terveystieto peruskoulun oppiaineeksi* [Health education should become a school subject]. *Suomen Lääkärilehti, 4,* 380-383.
26. Korhonen, J., Eloranta, T., & Santala, E. (1984). *Lukion terveystieto* [Health Education of the General Upper Secondary Education]. Keuruu: Otava.
27. Halila, A. (1949). *Suomen kansakoululaitoksen historia. Toinen osa* [The history of the Finnish educational system. Part II]. Turku: Uuden Auran osakeyhtiön kirjapaino.
28. Uusiautti, S., Paksuniemi, M., & Määttä, K. (2013). Elementary education and children's lives during the World War II in Finland. *Journal of Studies in Education, 3*(1), 84-102.
29. Paksuniemi, M., Uusiautti, S., & Määttä, K. (2012). Teetotalism as the core of education at the elementary school teacher training college of Tornio, Finland. *History of Education & Children's Literature, 7*(1), 389-411.
30. Cunningham, P., & Gardner, P. (1999). "Saving the nation's children": teachers, wartime evacuation in England and Wales and the construction of national identity. *History of Education, 28*(3), 327-337.
31. Grosvenor, I. (1999). "There's no place like home": education and the making of national identity. *History of Education, 28*(3), 235-250.
32. Growes, S., & Laws, C. (2000). Children's experience of physical education. *European Journal of Physical Education, 5*(1), 22-27.
33. Trost, S. G. (2006). Public health and physical education. In D. Kirk, D. MacDonald, & M. O'Sullivan (Eds.), *The handbook of physical education*. London: Sage.
34. Campbell, R. A. (2008). Making sober citizens: the legacy of indigenous alcohol regulation in Canada, 1777-1985. *Journal of Canadian Studies, 42*(1), 105-126.

34

35. Room, R. (1992). The impossible dream? Routes to reducing alcohol problems in a temperance culture. *Journal of Substance Abuse, 4*, 91-106.
36. Zimmerman, J. (1994). The dilemma of Miss Jolly: Scientific temperance and teacher professionalism, 1882-1904. *History of Education Quarterly, 34*, 413-431.
37. Albert, C., & Davia, M. A. (2010). Education is a key determinant of health in Europe: a comparative analysis of 11 countries. *Health Promotion International, 26*(2), 163-170.
38. Lindström, B., & Eriksson, M. (2011). From health education to healthy learning: implementing salutogenesis in educational science. *Scandinavian Journal of Public Health, 39*(suppl. 6), 85-92.
39. Morgan, A., & Haglund, B. J. (2009). Social capital does matter for adolescent health: evidence from the English HBSC study. *Health Promotion International, 24*(4), 363-372.
40. Rask, M., Määttä, K., & Uusiautti, S. (2013). The challenges of health education. *Problems of Education in the 21st Century, 51*, 91-103.
41. Tountas, Y., & Dimitrakaki, C. (2006). Health education for youth. *Pediatric Endocrinal Reviews, 3*, 222-225.
42. Kannas, L. (2005). Terveystieto-oppiaineen pedagogisia lähtökohtia. In H. Peltonen & L. Kannas (Eds.), *Terveystieto tutuksi – ensiapua terveystiedon opettamiseen* [Familiarize with health education – first aid to health education] (pp. 9-36). Helsinki: Hakapaino.
43. Hyry-Honka, O., Määttä, K., & Uusiautti, S. (2012). The role of health capital in health promotion. *International Journal of Health Promotion and Education, 50*(3), 125-134.
44. Williams, J. H. (2007). Teachers' perspectives of children's mental health service needs in urban elementary schools. *Children & Schools, 29*, 95-107.
45. Kickbusch, I. S. (2001). Health literacy: addressing the health and education divide. *Health Promotion International, 16*(3), 289-297.
46. Gerdtham, U.-G., Johannesson, M., Lundberg, L., & Isacson, D. (1999). The demand for health: results from new measures of health capital. *European Journal of Political Economy, 15*(3), 501-521.

Health Capital and Health Literacy as the Fundamental Health Skills

The Role of Health Capital in Health Promotion

Outi Hyry-Honka, Kaarina Määttä and Satu Uusiautti

You could ask any man or woman on the street to name the most important three things in their lives and one of their choices would be health. Everyone appreciates health and wishes they would stay healthy for their whole life span. What things does health consist of then? How can one cherish it? What promotes health? Are there some factors that one could gather in order to improve health and that would 'pay dividend'?

French sociologist Bourdieu[1,2] has analyzed the concept of capital and developed a theory of capital types. O'Rand[3] has furthered Bourdieu's thinking by adding the number of capital types and perspectives. Their work challenges researchers to look for other possible capital types that have already been brought out in various disciplines.

In this article, our aim is to develop a concept of health capital that would advance health promotion. The basis of this idea grounds on our research and teaching work that have focused on health promotion, the development of health education, and confronting challenges. Cherishing health creates a basis for happy life and positive human health. Furthermore, health promotion and preventing diseases require new research and approaches[4].

The first author of this article has written her doctoral thesis about middle school age youngsters' health resources[5], the second author has studied the preconditions for the development of youngsters' emotional life and balanced growth[6], and the third author has studied the keys to success at work[e.g.7]. Together, we have studied and defined—leaning on positive psychology—both good teacherhood[8], success at work and in life[9] as well as health promoting love for fellow humans in nursing[10].

Today's world sets a new spectrum of threats to people's health. Adults have to cope with the insecurity and stress, burnout and lassitude caused by rapidly changing modern working life: at the same time, for example, increasing unemployment and other societal problems pose demanding challenges for people's well-being and health. Furthermore, not only among adults but also among children and youngsters a variety of problems occurs: depression, exclusion, psychosocial problems, mental problems, and especially the increase in learning difficulties are worrying[see 11,12].

This tendency justifies or downright calls for a new kind of approach to health. Positive psychology presents one starting point for the kind of study on health that concentrates on human well-being and advances its occurrence[e.g.13]

However, the contemplation of health promotion has lacked a compiling framework [see 14]. Therefore, the aim of this article is to present such a theoretical framework. The purpose is to launch a new concept that we call health capital.

In this article, we introduce previous opinions and researches that have affected the birth and formation of the above-mentioned concept. Our approach leans on the theoretical analysis on previous research. First, we analyze the essence of health, its definition and research. Then, we will dissect the concept of capital. This review will result in the concept of health capital, the meaning and tenability of which we will evaluate in the end.

The Definition of Health and Health-related Research

Health has been reflected from various perspectives both in nursing science and sociology, psychology, the science of education, and other human sciences. Among other things, health covers taking care of oneself, committing oneself to treatment, and health-related choices[15]. In addition, health has been considered as an expression of the individualistic way of human being, inner strength or possibility, ability to use strengths and feeling good[5,16]. The concept of empowerment has been connected to health[17] when health has been regarded as human prowess and feeling of power. Health has also been associated with life management, well-being, and life course of a human being[16]. The most recent viewpoints are social capital[e.g. 18], cultural capital[e.g. 19], and health literacy[e.g. 20].

In the course of time, the concept of health has developed, diversified, and expanded. Nowadays, health is seen as a positive and comprehensive factor that belongs to people's entire circle and course of life and culture and which is connected to people's resources. Health is no longer considered a static state but a changing and dynamic learning or development process by its nature. Genotype, living conditions, learned and adopted information, skills, and attitudes affect health. What kind of experiences people get in order to promote their health influences their development greatly. This kind of comprehensive, multidimensional, dynamic, and contextual idea of health challenge research, teaching and health promotion activities[21].

The essence of health and health promotion can also be reviewed through resources[e.g. 22]. According to Antonovsky[23], resources can be divided into inner and outer resources that people use when pursuing advancing in their life in parallel with their goals. Based on Antonovsky's division, inner health resources can be defined consisting of the positive features and strengths that are inside a human being self. Whereas outer health resources consist of the health-related positive features and strengths in a human being's environment.

Health has been studied to a great extent from the point of view of preventing diseases. Thus, the interest has been on people's health-related habits and attitudes, ways of life, risk and problem behavior and how to change them. At the same time, health- related studies have concentrated on themes around one problem at a time, such as smoking[24], alcohol and drug abuse[25], violent behavior[26], eating disorders[27], dating and sex[6], stress[28], and so on; while a holistic and positive approach to health has been minimal.

Theoretical Introduction on the Concept of Capital

Initially, capital originates in classic economic science. In economics, capital is considered as one of the three factors of production in addition to a state and work. It can be utilized for producing other commodities, it is made by a human being and it is not used directly in a manufacturing process like raw materials. Investing means increasing capital. In order to be able to invest, it is necessary to create commodities that are not consumed immediately but used for producing other commodities[29]. Capital needs to meet certain criteria. It is a reserve that will be used when necessary, it is subject to consumption, and it can be gathered and invested in[30].

The Traditional Classification of Capital

Often, the contemplation of capital grounds on Bourdieu's[1] classification of capitals. According to his original theory, cultural capital, economic capital, and social capital form the capital types. The total amount and composition of cultural, economic, and social capital are factors that an individual can use as his/her resources in a competition situation[2]. Cultural capital refers to the ownership of cultural products, a certain way of life, and making choices as well as the ability to make use of and produce culture. There are three types of cultural capital: the aptitudes of mind and body aka capital incarnated as habitus; capital can be turned into objects or various cultural products such as books, pictures, or machinery; and capital institutionalized as qualifications.[see 31] An individual's education and capital are thus connected to cultural capital providing his/her with a good societal position. Parents affect the accumulation of their children's cultural capital. Parents' attitudes toward education and their own all-rounded education and educational level have influence on the nature of the cultural capital that a child gets. Economic capital consists of an individual's financial capital, possessions, and ownership (money, things, income, and wealth). It is the most concrete one of the capital types. Other capital types can be turned into economic capital under certain conditions.

Social and Symbolic Capital

When it comes to social capital, Bourdieu is interested in the competition for social capital in social markets and how others can collect more resources related to social capital than others. According to Bourdieu[1], social capital is the entity of those actual and potential resources that are connected to social relationships and the ability to mobilize people. Social capital can be institutionalized as a societal position that can also be turned into money[1]. Social capital does not have the same kind of incarnated or concretized existence as economic or cultural capital. Social capital is immaterial capital and is connected to mutual recognition and appreciation. Social capital is likely to decrease along with aging which, for its part, affects cultural and economic capital[32].

In Bourdieu's theory, the capitals are mainly composed of concrete things that can be gathered and that are, at least to some extent, objectively measurable. Capitals are slow and usually gathering them takes a long time. Capitals can be transmitted from one generation to another. The whole life means struggle over the control of various capitals[1,2].

Afterwards, Bourdieu added symbolic capital in his theory of capital types. It refers to an individual or people's ability and power to affect defining the value of other capitals (e.g. power affects the health conception of each moment). However, symbolic capital is not a capital type of its own but it is any type of capital or a qualification that changes into symbolically effective when people appreciate it. Symbolic capital is the power of determination and the value of other capitals depends on it. Furthermore, other capital types are parts of symbolic capital. For example, language tells about symbolic power. Symbolic capital relates to an individual's subjective experiences, feelings, or the value something has for an individual[1].

Life Course Capitals

In the field of societal and social sciences, the concept of capital has been linked to social equality and thus the purpose is to describe the division of social and economic resources within a society through the concept of capital. Accumulation can be uneven and cause social inequality between individuals or various population groups. O'Rand[3] specifies the concept of capital to cover the whole life span. Life course capital refers to a group of interconnected resources that enable increasing social equality and well-being. It increases or decreases along the life course when fulfilling human needs and hopes. Accumulation can be directed to a certain extent and evened by investing in social equality and well-being, for example by developing education or social and health services. O'Rand[3] distinguishes several different types of life course capitals. Partly, O'Rand's capital types are similar to Bourdieu's. However, O'Rand divided the capitals into individual-level and community-level capitals.

Individual-level capitals

According to O'Rand[3], human capital, personal capital, cultural capital, social capital, and psycho-physical capital comprise the individual-level capital. Human capital consists of such individual people's knowledge, skills, and characteristics that advance creating personal, social, and economic well-being. It also covers motivation, behavior, and the ability to learn new concepts. Human capital can be affected by an individual's upbringing, education, professional proficiency, and work experience. It is manifested through an individual's social roles and ability to handle difficult life situations and cope with stress. The core of personal capital lies in people's identity. Personal capital involves an individual's flexibility, positive emotions, self-confidence, opportunities to control his/her life, and life style. Personal capital combines people in their environment and community. Instead, cultural capital consists of language, interaction styles, and aesthetics[3].

In O'Rand's[3] thinking, social capital is the unity of direct and indirect social relationships that people can use when necessary. Social capital consists of family, friends, work and profession-related as well as communal and societal nets. As such, social capital is a group of non-economic resources with which a human being can achieve social status and well-being.

Psychophysical capital covers an individual's mental and physical health as well as mental and physical shape and durability[3]. Karisto and Konttinen[33] refer to the concept of energy capital and include health, performance, vitality, and self-image in it. Some researchers consider mental and physical health as a part of human capital[e.g. 34] and do not regard it as a capital type of its own like O'Rand does.

Some of the personal capital types diminish when used in the course of time (e.g. physical shape and durability in psychophysical capital), whereas some of them strengthen and increase (e.g. professional proficiency and competence in human capital). Various capital types are interconnected and they can strengthen each other[3].

Community-level capitals

In O'Rand's[3] theory, institutional capital (welfare-state-based benefits and public commodities), communal capital (local employment situation and service system), and moral capital (inter-generation solidarity, social identity, and affection) are the types of community-level capital. Therefore, the concept of capital refers to personal, communal, and societal features, operational resources and possibilities, which enable people to acquire new things, act in various environments and contexts, and execute economic and societal activities.

What is Health Capital?

Some researchers say that capital consists of the entity of resources. For example, Coleman[35] defines social capital as a total of resources that have become concentrated within the social structure. O'Rand[3], for his part, refers to the reserve of resources that is gathered along the course of life and covers a variety of areas of life, as life course capital does. According to the researchers, those areas of life where resources exist are economic, social, cultural—historical, human, and personal area.

Because health and health promotion lean greatly on resources, we ended up combining health resources with the concept of capital. These connecting viewpoints gave birth to the concept of health capital. This contemplation deepens and adapts capital theories and develops the conceptualization of health promotion further by contributing a new way of dissecting it. Figure 1 illustrates the position of health capital in relation to other capital types. Health capital is the entity of health-related resources where crucial factors are inner and outer health resources. Health capital is not considered equal to other capital types[see 3,33] nor is it included solely inside human capital[see 34]. Health capital is regarded as a part of other capital types leaning on O'Rand's[3] idea according to which every capital type relates directly or indirectly to health.

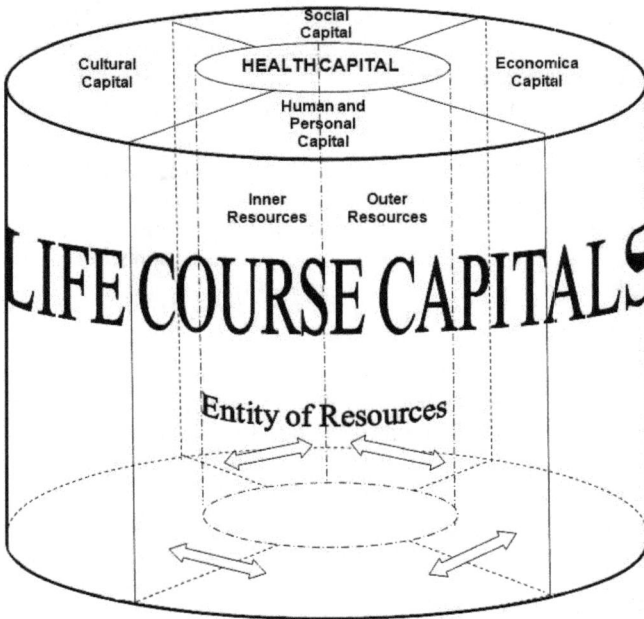

Figure 1. The interconnectedness of health capital with other capital types. [see 5, p. 31]

Health capital forms a part of human or personal capital to the extent that people's knowledge, skills, and learning are connected to health. Skills that relate to health directly or indirectly are for example the ability to take care of oneself, health literacy, interaction, self-assessment, and problem-solving skills as well as the ability to handle things related to becoming seriously ill. This area also involves people's mental and physical shape, durability, and performance. Health capital is a part of social capital when human relationships and nets support people's health, security, and well-being. Health capital is a part of cultural capital when it comes to respecting health, health ideologies, and health-related habits and customs. In the field of economic capital, health capital refers to the resources, machinery, tools, and facilities available for promoting people's mental and physical shape and health.

People need sufficient health capital in order to be able to make relevant choices concerning their health and life and to promote their health. The more people have health resources, the stronger health capital they have and the better they are able to maintain and promote their health. The less people have health resources, the weaker their health capital is and the harder they will find maintaining and promoting their health when the risk of becoming ill increases.

Together the capital types form a reserve of resources that make people strong and powerful. With this reserve, an individual can control and direct his/her living conditions consciously and have an influence on what happens to him/her.

The concept of health capital is new and is mentioned only in very few articles and textbooks. Shim[36] uses the concept of 'cultural health capital' and connects it with health care. Kunnari[37] mentions the concept or 'the experience-based capital of physical exercise' when analyzing the connection between physical exercise with especially the area of health and self-development. Among others, Åhlberg[34] refers to the concept of health capital. Health capital is an important part of human capital that is worth taking care of. However, the above-mentioned researchers fail to define the concept in detail and they do not connect it with its wider contexts. According to O'Rand[3], it would be important to notice the contents and relationships between capitals.

Criticism on Health Capital

The new concepts of capital have been criticized abundantly and their implementation always involves some risks. Criticism originates in the thought that the traditional concept of capital can be defined unambiguously and has established its context of use. The new concepts of capital mix up the conceptual clarity. According to Hjerppe[30], capital is a reserve that can be used when necessary; it can be spent, increased, and invested in.

These criteria are utilized here for evaluating the concept of health capital. In order to be capital, health capital has to be a reserve that an individual can intentionally use to realize his/her health-related intentions. One has to be able to gather capital and invest in it. It is, for example, possible to increase health capital for the part of health-related knowledge, skills, and expertise as well as physical and mental shape[38]. In addition, the original concept of capital involves a thought that it has to be subject to consuming. For example, physical performance is consumed, decreases along with aging, but on the other hand, in a short run, physical performance becomes weak if it is not taken care of or used for example by exercising[37].

Health capital does not meet all criteria for capital strictly; which is the case with other immaterial capitals (e.g. human capital, personal capital, and social capital) as well. If the fact that health capital makes people's action easier by improving their health (in other words, is a resource that makes profit) is considered sufficient, it is capital. Health capital enables for its part economic action and is therefore a felicitous expression in relation to the original use. Good health and health capital bring economic profit for people by enabling them to work and perform and spare them from the costs related to illnesses and treatments. From the societal perspective, national health has a great meaning. Good national health secures the supply and stability of work force and spares tax revenues to other uses. However, health and health capital cannot be considered important only for economic profit[39]. They also enable versatile self-fulfillment.

Expanding the use of the concept of capital involves other dangers than just turning the concept ambiguous. Health capital can become instrumental or suffer from inflation. Health and health capital can be pursued only because something else, for example economic wealth can be achieved with them and thus its intrinsic value and absolute nature disappear. A negative consequence may also be that every activity that makes functioning easier will be called capital when the concept loses its explanatory strength[see 40, p. 30-33]. The concept of health capital can be clarified by distinguishing the sources, approximate concepts, and implications of health capital with each other[41], when the approximate concepts and health that are measurable at least to some extent would represent the actual health capital, and health would be the consequence of health capital.

Discussion

For all the criticism presented in the conclusion, the use of health capital seems justified. Health capital is an important adjunct to the other life course capitals. The concept completes Bourdieu's and O'Rand's ways of dissecting capitals. Health capital partly includes the same elements as Bourdieu's and O'Rands capital types. However, health makes its content specific. Defining inner and outer resources as health resources when people use them to promote their health and defining health capital as the entity of health resources and as a part of other capital types offer a comprehensive theoretical framework for contemplating health promotion and a new viewpoint to resource-based health- promotion work.

Defining health capital as capital is reasonable also because the concept of capital is positively charged. Capital is something that is worth acquiring and investing in. Therefore, using the concept of health capital can, for its part, increase the appreciation of health[5]. It is meaningful also for the development of nursing education.

Especially, thinking of health capital and recognizing health capital are important for the young. They spend a remarkable part of their time and everyday life at school. Therefore, youngsters' experiences at school and activities that strengthen youngsters' health resources at the school community contribute to their overall development and health. In addition to health education, many other subjects at school and the school for its outer settings transmit the health-related knowledge, skills, attitudes, and values[42]. At its best, school can strengthen determinedly and systematically youngsters' health resources and increase their health capital. It will reflect in youngsters' ability to live as citizens who cherish and promote their health.

In order for the school to function in a manner that promotes youngsters' health, health perspective has to be noticed comprehensively in all teaching activities, not just health education and other school activities. Teachers' readiness for supporting health promotion should be taken care of by providing them with opportunities for in-service education. Furthermore, it would be worth deliberating whether special health pedagogy should be developed to secure the implementation of health perspective in teaching[5].

The young can be engaged in health promotion by noticing their point of view. Their voices have to be listened to. Active youngsters create an active school where the common goal is the good health capital of the members of school community. Supporting youngsters' health and its promotion should be carried out systematically in the everyday life at school[see 5].

To be able to strengthen youngsters' resources and health capital with various actions, we have to know what factors are relevant especially from the point of view of the young. Their health resources and health capital remain potential until we have information about what they are and how much the young have them. In addition, we need to have consensus on the goal for attaining which resources and health capital are needed. Therefore, empirical testing of the concept of health capital is important in future.

References

1. Bourdieu, P. (1986). The forms of capital. In J. G. Richardson (Ed.), *Handbook of theory and research for sociology of education* (pp. 241-258). New York, NY: Greenwood Press.

46

2. Bourdieu, P. (1990). *Distinction. A social critique of the judgement of taste.* New York, NY: Routledge & Kegan Paul.
3. O'Rand, A. M. (2006). Stratification and the life course: life-course capital, life course risks, and social inequality. In R. Binstock & L. George (Eds.), *Handbook of aging and the social sciences* (pp. 145-162). Boston, MA: Academic Press.
4. Thorlindsson, T. (2010). Bring in the social context: towards an integrated approach to health promotion and prevention. *Scandinavian Journal of Public Health, 39*(16), 19–25.
5. Hyry-Honka, O. (2008). *Terveyspääoma kouluyhteisössä seitsemäsluokkalaisten käsitysten valossa* [Health capital in a school community as described by seventh graders]. (PhD Diss., University of Lapland, Rovaniemi, Finland.)
6. Määttä, K. (2010). How to learn to guide the young to love. *Educational Sciences and Psychology, 2*(17), 47–53.
7. Uusiautti, S., & Määttä, K. (2010). What kind of employees become awarded as Employees of the Year in Finland? *Enterprise and Work Innovation Studies, 6*, 53-73.
8. Määttä, K., & Uusiautti, S. (2011). Pedagogical love and good teacherhood. *In Education, 17*(2). http://ineducation.ca/article/pedagogical-love-and-good-teacherhood
9. Uusiautti, S., & Määttä, K. (2012). The successful combination of work and family in Finland: The ability to compromise as a key factor. *Journal of Comparative Family Studies, 43*(2), 151-163.
10. Paldanius, A., & Määttä, K. (2011). What are students' views of (loving) caring in nursing education in Finland? *International Journal of Caring Sciences, 4*(2), 81–89.
11. Bhatia, S. K., & Bhatia, S. C. (2007). Childhood and adolescent depression. *American Family Physician, 75*(1), 73–80.
12. Williams, J. H. (2007). Teachers' perspectives of children's mental health service needs in urban elementary schools. *Children & Schools, 29*(2), 95–107.
13. Aspinwall, L. G., & Tedeschi, R. G. (2010). The value of positive psychology for health psychology: a progress and pitfalls in examining the relation of positive phenomena to health. *Annals of Behavioral Medicine, 39*(1), 4–15.
14. Fitzpatrick, R. (2000). Measurement issues in health-related quality of life: challenges for health psychology. *Psychology and Health, 15*(1), 99–108.
15. Kickbusch, I. (1989). Self-care in health promotion. *Social Science & Medicine, 29*(2), 125–130.
16. Bech, P. (2003). Measuring well-being rather than the absence of distress symptoms: a comparison of the SF-36 mental health subscale and the WHO-five well-being scale. *International Journal of Methods in Psychiatric Research, 12*(2), 85–91.
17. Falk-Rafael, A. R. (2001). Empowerment as a process of evolving consciousness: a model of empowered caring. *Advances in Nursing Science, 18*(2), 25–32.
18. Morrow, V. (2004). Children's "social capital": Implications for health and well-being. *Health Education, 104*(4), 211–225.
19. Abel, T. (2008). Cultural capital and social inequality in health. *Journal of Epidemiology & Community Health, 62*(7), 627–633.
20. Nutbeam, D. (2008). The evolving concept of health literacy. *Social Science & Medicine, 67*, 2072–2078.
21. Albert, C., & Davia, M. A. (2011). Education is a key determinant of health in Europe: A comparative analysis of 11 countries. *Health Promotion International, 26*(29), 163–170.
22. Lindström, B., & Eriksson, M. (2011). From health education to healthy learning: Implementing salutogenesis in educational science. *Scandinavian Journal of Public Health, 39*(6), 85–99.

47

23. Antonovsky, A. (1996). The salutogenic model as a theory to guide health promotion. *Health Promotion International, 11*(1), 11–18.
24. Carver, V. (2003). Adolescents' attitudes and self-perceptions about anti-tobacco advocacy. *Health Education Research, 18*(4), 453–460.
25. Gitlow, S. (2006). *Substance use disorders: A practical guide.* Philadelphia, PA: Lippincott Williams and Wilkins.
26. Cooper, W. (2003). Planning of youth violence. Prevention programs: Development of a guiding measure. *Public Health Nursing, 20*(6), 432–439.
27. Dalle Grave, R. (2003). School-based prevention programs for eating disorders: Achievement and opportunities. *Disease Management & Health Outcomes, 11*(9), 579–593.
28. Chiesa, A., & Serretti, A. (2009). Mindfulness-based stress reduction for stress management in healthy people: A review and meta-analysis. *Journal of Alternative and Complementary Medicine, 15*(5), 593–600.
29. Dillard, D. (1982). Rewriting the principles of economics. *Journal of Economic Issues, 16*(2), 577–590.
30. Hjerppe, R. (1997). Sosiaalinen pääoma – tutkimisen arvioinen käsite [Social capital – a concept worth researching]. *Hyvinvointikatsaus, 1*(97), 26–29.
31. Lamont, M., & Lareau, A. (1988). Cultural capital: Allusions, gaps and glissandos in recent theoretical developments. *Sociological Theory, 6,* 153–168.
32. Marin, M. (2001). Successful ageing – Dependent on cultural and social capital? Reflections from Finland. *Indian Journal of Gerontology, 15*(1&2), 145–159.
33. Karisto, A., & Konttinen, R. (2004). *Kotiruokaa, kotikatua, kaukomatkailua* [Home food, home street, far-off travelling]. Helsinki: Palmenia.
34. Åhlberg, M. (2005). *YK:n kestävää kestävää kehitystä edistävän kasvatuksen vuosikymmen (2005–2014) biologian ja kestävän kehityksen didaktiikan sekä opettajan työn näkökulmasta* [The decade (2005–2014) of education promoting UN's sustainable development from the point of view of biology and didactics of sustainable development and teachers' work]. http://www.bulsa.helsinki.fi/ ~ maahlber/Ahlberg_Natu
35. Coleman, J. S. (1988). Social capital in the creation of human capital. *American Journal of Sociology, 94,* S95–S120.
36. Shim, J. K. (2010). Cultural health capital. A theoretical approach to understanding health care interactions and the dynamics of unequal treatment. *Journal of Health and Social Behavior, 51*(1), 1–15.
37. Kunnari, A. (2011). *Liikuntapääoma ja holistinen ihmiskä sitys liikuntaa opettavan työssä* [The experience-based capital of physical exercise and the holistic conception of human being in PE teachers' work]. (PhD Diss., University of Lapland, Rovaniemi, Finland.)
38. Adkins, N. R., & Corus, C. (2009). Health literacy for improved health outcomes: effective capital in the marketplace. *The Journal of Consumer Affairs, 43*(2), 199–222.
39. Abel, T. (2011). Money is not enough: exploring the impact of social and cultural resources on youth health. *Scandinavian Journal of Public Health, 390*(6), 57–71.
40. Ruuskanen, P. (2001). *Sosiaalinen pääoma – käsitteet, suuntaukset ja mekanismit* [Social capital – concepts, trends and mechanisms]. Helsinki: GIER.
41. Hyyppä, M. (2004). Kertyykö sosiaalisesta pääomasta kansanterveyttä? [Does social capital increase national health?] *Yhteiskuntapolitiikka, 69*(4), 380-386.
42. Tountas, Y., & Dimitrakaki, C. (2006). Health education for youth. *Pediatric Endocrinal Reviews, 3*(1), 222–225.

The Concept of the Experience-Based Capital of Physical Exercise (ECPE)

Ari Kunnari, Kaarina Määttä and Satu Uusiautti

Physical education is concentrated on studying the exercising body and ignored the experiential world, the human being as a holistic bodily, experiencing, and living exerciser[1]. In the Finnish school system, the aim of physical education is to provide such knowledge, skills, and experiences[2] based on which one may adopt a sporty lifestyle. But what are these experiences and how are they defined? What do the versatile experiences of physical exercise consist of?

In this article we introduce a theoretical model that was built based on the findings from a phenomenological study of the meanings of physical exercise and that introduces the concept of the experience-based capital of physical experience (ECPE)[see 3]. The research method was based on Giorgi's[4,5] and Perttula's[6,7] ways of implementing phenomenological research. The purpose of the original study was to find out what kinds of experiences PE-teachers gain from their work. The original study on which this article grounds on was carried out was a two-phase, qualitative studied conducted among 15 PE-teacher students at the Faculty of Education, University of Lapland, Finland[see 3]. First, they were asked to write essays about their experiences on physical exercise. In the second phase, the same participants were interviewed. The interview method was a phenomeno-logical interview[see 8,9] and the purpose was to get deeper information about their experiences. As a conclusion, a theoretical framework that illustrates the experiential world of physical exercise as one form of cultural capital was created.

In this article, the concept of the experiencebased capital of physical exercise (ECPE) will be introduced and analyzed. Furthermore, its connection with physical exercise and sport, and previous studies in the field are discussed. Bourdieu's cultural types will be reviewed which forms the basis of the concept of ECPE. Finally, the usability and offering of the concept not only for analyzing but also providing experiences of physical exercise in a more versatile manner will be evaluated.

Research on Physical Exercise

The body of studies of physical exercise is abundant: physical exercise and learning is studied for example from the perspectives of motor learning and control, and learning of exercising skills[10,11] but by developing various definitions of motor learning as well[12,13,14,15,17].Furthermore, there are studies about the connection between physical education and health[18,19]. Along research on physical education, some studies are focused on pupils' experiences on physical education[20,21,22,23] or on providing information that would support PE teaching[24].

Teachers' activity greatly affects experiences of physical education[25]. Therefore, the motivational atmosphere as a part of physical exercise and physical education has gained a foothold in research[26,27,28]. Although research on pupils' experiences-and partly on teachers' experiences as well-is abundant, the entity of experiences related to physical exercise has not been sketched or defined from the point of view of learning and subject matter. The purpose of this study is to contribute to this discussion by providing a new point of view by drawing parallels between physical exercise and the concept of capital.

The Concept of Capital

Initially, capital originates in classic economic science but is adopted in human sciences as well. According to O'Rand[29], the concept of capital covers the whole course of life. Karisto and Konttinen[30] use the concept of energy capital that includes health, ability to function, vitality, and self-image. Hyry-Honka[31] defines the concept of health capital as a part of the entity of resources and the sum of outer and inner health[see 3]. Hyry-Honka regards health capital as a part of other capital types (Bourdieu, O'Rand) leaning on O'Rand's view according to which all capital types are either directly or indirectly connected to health.

Bourdieu[32] divided capital into three types: cultural capital, economic capital, and social capital. The total amount and composition of cultural, economic, and social capital are factors that an individual can use as his or her resources[33].

a. Economic capital consists of an individual's financial capital, possessions and ownership (money, things, income, and wealth). It is the most concrete one of the capital types.

b. Cultural capital refers to the ownership of cultural products, a certain way of life and making choices as well as the ability to make use of and produce culture. An individual's education and capital are thus connected to cultural capital.

c. Social capital is the entity of those actual and potential resources that are connected to social relationships and the ability to mobilize people. Social capital does not have the same kind of incarnated or concretized existence than economic or cultural capital. Social capital is immaterial capital and is connected to mutual recognition and appreciation.

The concept of habitus is closely related to capitals. Bourdieu[34] defines habitus as an internalized structure that is common to all members of the same class; the schemas of observation, concepts, and actions that form the framework for common understanding and observation. De France[35] sees habitus as a universal description of how an individual participates and acts within the social world. All in all, habitus refers to the way of human existence and is an individual's experience-based way of action and take his or her environment. Social status has an influence on habitus, too.

Of Bourdieu's capital types, especially cultural capital is an interesting object to study. Bourdieu[36] considers sport as a part of cultural capital and also states that it functions as a factor that separates social classes from each other. Shilling[37], on the other hand, uses the concept of physical capital and argues that it cannot be seen just a part of cultural capital. Shilling[38] connects the concept with situated action to

> illustrate how the relationship between social field and physical capital can result in not only a continuation of habitual action—but in action informed by crisis and revelation—that can aid our understanding of the education of bodies. (p. 473)

In Bourdieuan thinking, capital seems to represent, first and foremost, a quality or a characteristic. Thus, various capital types represent a human being's different characteristics. These capital types are partly inherited in the form of rearing or heritage but partly they are acquired from outside the family, too[See 39]. According to Bourdieu[40], there are three states of cultural capital: the embodied state, such as long-lasting characteristics of the mind and body as a part of habitus; the objectified state, such as cultural goods; and the institutionalized state which Bourdieu calls a form of objectification.

In order to understand the concept of ECPE, it is crucial to perceive cultural capital especially from an individual's point of view: what belongs to an individual's cultural capital and how the capital is constructed. Being different from the economic and social capital, cultural capital consists of socially distinguishing tastes, knowledge, skills, and acts that are objectified to cultural products and embody as implicit practical knowledge, skills, and natures. These, on the other hand, are expressed as emotions, thinking, and action that Bourdieu calls habitus[40]. Cultural capital is commonly described via education and school success. Dumais[41] points out, however, that there is no consensus on the meaning of cultural capital. Although Bourdieu emphasizes how cultural capital is transmitted from parents to children, the purpose here is not to discuss cultural capital from to point of view of the separation between social classes[e.g.42]. Instead, the interest is focused on how and on what grounds ECPE could form a part of cultural capital and what ECPE consists of. Along the life-span, people collect and get knowledge, skills, tastes, and preferences in every areas of life-at home, at school and further education, in leisure activities and hobbies. Therefore, cultural capital cannot only be regarded as one's level of education.

Recent studies[e.g. 42,43,44,45] have determinedly aimed at testing Bourdieu's opinion on sport functioning as cultural capital. Generally, research results support the finding. Bourdieu[36] himself points out that the likelihood to have certain sport as a hobby depends a social class and the possibility of achieving the aesthetic and austere dispositions related to the sport as they are regarded as a part of that particular sport. This brings us back at the concept of habitus. According to Bourdieu[40], differences in life-styles and participation in sports partly depend on various habituses. On the other hand, they are manifestations of various cultural and social capitals and vice versa. Light[46] considers habitus a personal product of one's life history and social experiences. Therefore, ECPE as the manifesttation of experiences of physical exercise could partly construct cultural capital.

Bourdieu[36] also employs the concept of physical capital to refer a form of cultural capital that is manifested as a physical skill, power, ways of exercising, etc. Then, physical capital is an extremely bodily phenomenon and capital that can be turned into, for example, economic capital (e.g. sport may become an occupation). According to Välipakka[47], physical capital is cultural capital and its production occurs in relation to those habits that are invested in body. By dissecting physical exercise as everyday action, it is possible consider physical capital merely as a life-long process.

Bourdieu's classification of capitals provides an explicit framework for constructing the content of ECPE whereas in O' Rand's categorization of capitals, ECPE would form a part of several capital types. Bourdieu offers an opportunity to consider ECPE as its own entity but simultaneously constructing an individual's cultural capital. The concept of ECPE means capital that is acquired through exercising experiences and that we understand as a form of the embodied state of cultural capital. It appears as ways of action and aptitudes. Therefore, ECPE is not corresponding to economic capital, nor does it produce social capital as such. Instead, habitus as one of Bourdieu's key concepts and as a human being's way of expressing cultural capital is an important concept in ECPE: Could ECPE be expressed through habitus as well?

The Experience-Based Capital of Physical Exercise (ECPE)

Theory

Based on above-mentioned premises in Bourdieu's classification of capitals, experiences of physical exercise can be considered stakes that actors on the field try to gather. The geography of ECPE as a part of Bourdieu's capital types is illustrated in Figure 1. Social and capital partly determine what kinds of experiences one can possibly get (the school, distractions, parents' aptitude for sports, etc.). As the experiences of physical exercises accumulate, one develops one's own ECPE that possibly directs one's sportive hobbies or attitude toward physical exercise.

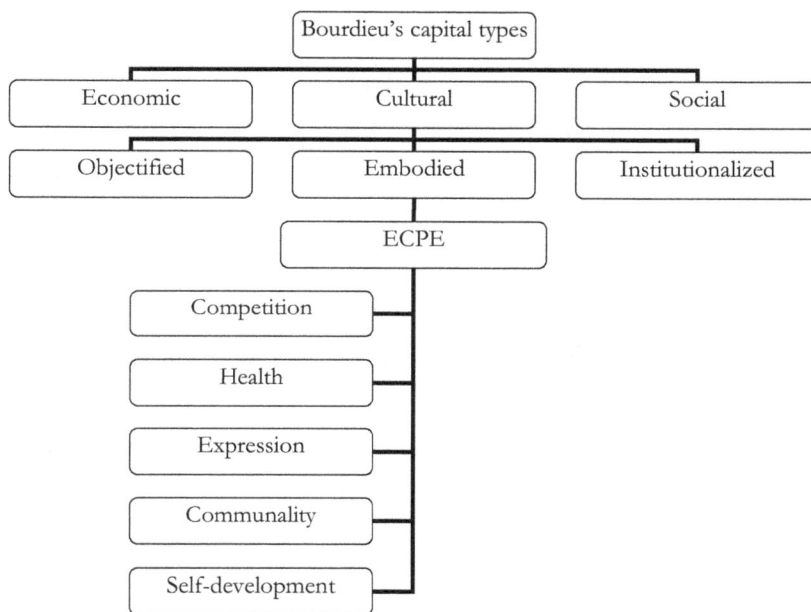

Figure 1. ECPE as a part of cultural capital in Bourdieu's classification of capitals.

However, the nature of experiences that lay the foundation of the capital is multi-dimensional and therefore, the content of ECPE can differ from a person to another and thus, the theoretical starting point is that one or some of the fields of ECPE become dominant. Next, we will briefly introduce these fields of ECPE (see also Figure 1) and then discuss and compare it with other relevant categorizations.

The fields of ECPE are competition, health, expression, communality, and self-development.

1. Competition as a field of ECPE has its meaning through victory or loss. The experience may be either a victory or loss over some other or oneself and relate to the feeling of superiority or inferiority. The capital of competition may partly consist of experiences that define the status or value within a community or circle of acquaintances.

2. People do not do physical exercise just to win but also to keep up health. Health can be defined in two different ways: preventing illnesses and mobility which also includes physical shape. When experiences on physical exercise are mostly health-related experiences, the question is about the field of health in ECPE. The experience may also represent the field of health when it brings pleasure and delight (or resentment).

3. Physical exercise may also be experienced so that the body is primarily considered as the channel of expression. The experience may originate in the ways one is able to express various things through one's body or body movement. Body may be used for expressing or bringing the spectator various moods or ethical or aesthetic experiences. The experience results from the success of expressing oneself to others or how others take the expression. Recognizing and accepting one's own body movements may bring about moods that form the field of expression in ECPE.
4. The field of communality increases ECPE when the meaning of physical exercise originates in living, experiencing, and doing together. Belonging to a group, the importance of group activity and shared playing are emphasized. Furthermore, spurring others or received support and spur from others belong to this category.
5. The pure experience of physical exercise that gets its meaning as understanding and realizations increases the capital that provides people with the skills and knowledge to mental self-development. Instead of just exploring the limits of physical performance [e.g. 48,49], this field of ECPE refers to actual capability to do; so-called soul-searching. For one cannot do conscious soul-searching without having developed proper tools for it. Therefore, this category is called the field of self-development.

The above-mentioned categorization of ECPE grounds on Klemola's[48] physical exercise projects. Klemola divided these projects into four based on the primary purpose of physical exercise. They are physical exercise as the project of victory, health, expression, and self. Physical exercise projects do not represent strictly just one of the above-mentioned project types. What project is in question depends on its meaning for the one who does physical exercise. Klemola studied physical exercise projects so that each project appears the best in the form of some particular sport: for example, the project of victory in competitive sports, the project of health in keep-fit, the project of expression in dancing, and the project of self in budo sport.

Projects are not, however, sufficient reasoning for ECPE. A project as a word describes merely a process, doing, or experiences that an individual gathers form ECPE. The idea of ECPE is grounded on the phenomenological chance of pure experience[e.g. 50] and the interpretative nature of ECPE. Pure experience refers to an experience that lacks any natural attitude. In other words, the experience or the quality of the experience has not been pre-determined but the experience is "pure" in this sense. Although no one cannot know whether the experience can appear in the above-mentioned manner in practice; consequently, it merely forms a philosophical basis when considered from the phenomenological perspective. The way individuals experience physical exercise can vary regardless of the initial purpose of the physical exercise. Therefore, it is possible to categorize experiences based on the way they appear to individuals for experience may represent any field of the capital depending on what sport one does or what was the purpose of doing physical exercise. The principled difference is that in Klemola's project thinking physical exercise is understood through the project and the project, thus, functions as the pre-understanding about the meanings of physical exercise. According to Husserl's thinking, a project should, in that case, be the prevailing horizon which would be difficult to alter because experience gained from physical exercise would always be in accordance with the horizon.

Bourdieu states that various forms of capital are people's characteristics. Given this idea, various fields of ECPE may be regarded as characteristics in which one may direct his or her sportive activities. Experiences gained from physical exercise may, however, belong to any field of ECPE regardless of the sport. Therefore, ECPE is a horizon which is interpreted based on the experiences gained from physical exercise. ECPE may direct the sport hobby or the form of exercising but it does not direct the experience had on physical exercise. Thus, ECPE (the horizon) is easier to change its form (to be interpreted differently). Someone who does some ball games at the competition level makes a good example. When doing physical exercise, he or she is either at a competition or training. Thus, physical exercise would have its meaning based on the fact whether he or she is able to develop or whether the game is won or lost. According to the idea of ECPE, one may have other kinds of experiences as well. It might be that the topmost experience in the game or training may be related to how the performances look like. On the other hand, one may find physical exercise an aid for a headache after reading for an exam. Then, the topmost experience would represent the health among the fields of ECPE. ECPE is not connected to some sport but it is the capital of everyone's personal experience on physical exercise.

Evaluating the Concept of the Experience-Based Capital of Physical Exercise

It is worth critically dissecting the concept of ECPE. ECPE is a metaphoric concept similar to social capital. Therefore, it is difficult to draw conclusions with it. It can be partly difficult to understand how the concepts of capital and the presumption of "non-existence of social classes" can be molded within the point of view of personal experiences. Yet, cultural capital is a capital of its own in relation to other capitals. One essential aspect in cultural capital is power. Could ECPE be, however, property? Traditionally, capital is the means of exchange whereas someone's property does not have to be valuable to others. According to[51] criteria, capital is, however, a reserve that can be used when necessary. Capital, when considered in this way, can decrease (be spent), and be gathered and invested in. ECPE does not meet these criteria fully when it comes to the conditions of being used when necessary or decreasing. Instead, ECPE is merely unconscious as it directs action and can possibly alter along new experiences.

Bourdieu's classification explicitly brings out the differences between social classes. It is not directly included in the concept of ECPE but merely indirectly via the concept of habitus. According to this theory, one or some fields of ECPE can become dominant. Then, ECPE is partly manifested through an individual's habitus. Bourdieu's starting point is that members of the same social class have similar habitus. This notion would mean that populations, professions, or other communities could also be analyzed within the framework of ECPE. For example, it is worth asking whether PE teacher training produces some sort of common capital of physical experience. Or do people with similar ECPE tend to become PE teachers and, if this is the case, do they share some kind of a group habitus typical of PE teachers?

It is relevant to assess the concept of ECPE in the light of research on the meanings of physical exercise. Zacheus[52] studied the importance of different types of physical exercise perceived by Finnish adolescents (under 20-year-olds). As a result of his factor analysis, 11 entities were formed: competition, health/well-being, physicality, sociality, relaxation, fashion, masculinity, mental growth, lonely toil, parents' expectations, and economic affordability. It is interesting to compare Zacheus's categorization with the fields of ECPE. Competition is found in both of them. Health/well-being and physicality represent the field of health. The social factor resembles the field of communality. Masculinity and fashion appear similar to the field of expression. Relaxation and mental growth correspond to the idea of self-development. Although the rest three categories do not fit in the fields of ECPE, the factors are, as a rule, in line with the concept.

Koski and Tähtinen[53] studied the meanings based on which the youth build their relationship with physical exercise. The researchers found seven dimensions: competition and target-orientation, health and physical shape, joy and play, sociality, soul-searching, growth and development, and sport-specific meanings. Lehmuskallio[54] described the most important cultural meanings in school-age children's physical exercise habits. The ranking order was the following: (1) comfort and good mood, (2) family-centeredness and physicality, (3) extreme, (4) appetite for success, (5) and superficiality. In the above-mentioned studies including the field of ECPE, the entities of meanings, that are the categories, are somewhat similar although they have different names and partly different contents. The similarities in these categorizations become visible when they are dissected in the form of a table (see Table 1).

Table 1. Five categorizations of the meanings of physical exercise [by retelling 47,53,55,56,57,58]

Renson I	Renson II	Eichberg	Klemola	Honkonen & Suoranta	The fields of ECPE
A Instrumental	A A British sport	A Performance	A The project of victory	A Intensive training	A Competition
physical culture, physical performance sport	*success, performance, competition*				*in relation to others and oneself, the position*
	B Swedish gymnastics	B A health tool	B The project of health	B Health speech	*B* Health
	health				*feelings, physical shape, health, diversity*
C Autotelic	C Traditional frolic			C Entertainment	
Plays, games	*Joy, being together*				
D Expressive	D A performance sport	D Bodily experience	D The project of expression		D Expression
performance dancing		*expression, experientality*			*the way it appears, is expressed*
	E German turner			E Socialization	E Communality
	education, group activity				*the group, games, shared activity, spur*
			F The project of self		F Self-development
					developing spirituality and knowledge

ECPE differs in two significantly different ways from other five categorizations represented in Table 1 which presents a summary of the meanings of the offering and tradition of physical exercise. As can be seen in the table, there are plenty of similarities between the categorizations. However, the reasoning of ECPE grounds on the assumption that experience is a pure experience and intuition without the pre-determined influence of the social world of physical exercise. The starting point is that a human being could experience physical exercise without Husserl's reference to the natural attitude. The meaning of physical exercise can represent any field of ECPE and thus construct the horizon of ECPE. ECPE can itself direct one's attitude to various sports and the way one does physical exercise. A human being's social and economic capital affect what kinds of situations and sportive hobbies one can participate in. They do not, however, affect the meaning physical exercise has within the framework of ECPE.

Another significant difference originates in the research approach and research setting. Three of the studies (Koski and Tähtinen's, Zacheus's, and Lehmuskallio's study) introduced in this article were based on large data and reported with quantitative measures. In other studies, entities were formed based on predetermined sum variables. The fields of ECPE were found out by familiarizing with the meanings elicited through the phenomenological method. Thus, the meanings are brought out as the participants describe them.

Based on the previous, the idea of ECPE and its fields seem justified and even comprehensive. It is noteworthy that the fields of ECPE were created before familiarizing with the studies presented in Table 1 and other analyses.

Discussion

An important purpose of this article was to introduce a theoretical model for outlining the experience of physical exercise in a versatile manner. The theory creates a way of thinking and an apparatus for analyzing the world according to a specific theoretical framework. Yet, the framework is constructed based on meanings and entities of meanings driven from the authentic data.

A diversified conceptualization of physical exercise provides an opportunity to analyze ECPE from the perspective of the supply of physical exercise. If experiences of physical exercise are considered stakes in the field along with Bourdieu's idea, the fields of the capital of physical education make a tool for providing versatile experiences through which one can acquire as wide ECPE as possible.

Although the idea of ECPE and the related concept of habitus can be a way of studying the reserve of experiences among various groups of population, age cohorts, or professions, we want to highlight how the idea of ECPE could be used in physical education. When ECPE is considered an interpretative horizon, the basis of physical education could be the fields of ECPE. The concept of the horizon helps and makes it easier to perceive ECPE as changing which makes it a functional starting point and even a practical tool for the planning of teaching and how the educational event and the relationship with the student are constructed. As ECPE may alter, the starting point for educational planning may be input/output –thinking where the goal of action is Introducing the Concept of the Experience-Based Capital of Physical Exercise (ECPE) to provide experiences in a certain, predetermined field of ECPE. The practical action itself may still take place within sports education but the goals of action may be different.

Education that grounds on the idea of ECPE can be planned in three different ways. First, the starting point can be how various sports increase ECPE. Second, the planning can be focused on how to include within one sport such action and situations that enable the accumulation of all-round ECPE. Third-and this might support the best the accumulation of ECPE as pure experience-the starting point could be to think how teaching could cross the limits of sports. According to Koski and Tähtinen[53], various forms of physical exercise, such as different sports, are filled with specific expectations based on which people define their relationship to sports. Various forms of physical exercise can be experienced in a more diversified manner if they are approached without sport-specific contents.

In this article, the philosophical starting point to ECPE lies in the possibility of pure experience. The focus is, thus, how to provide individual people with as a versatile world of experiences of physical exercise as possible. The five fields of ECPE and the entities of meanings involved are the answer. Sketches on the accumulation of PE-teachers' ECPE that are drawn so far were based on interviews. Preliminary research results appeared interesting. It seemed that the participants perceived those fields of ECPE significant that also were the most dominant in them. Furthermore, it seemed to affect the ways the PE-teachers carried out PE education and how they confronted and perceived the exercising student. Given this important notion, more studies in order to develop a suitable and practical indicator to measure ECPE is needed as it could be useful to analyzing and developing PE education.

References

1. Talbott, M. (1997). Kohti kokemuksen tutkimista? [Toward research on experience?] *Liikunta & Tiede, 4*, 22–23.
2. *The National Core Curriculum for Basic Education 2004.* (2004) Helsinki: Finnish National Board of Education.
3. Kunnari, A. (2011). *Liikuntapääoma ja holistinen ihmiskäsitys liikuntaa opettavan työssä* [The experience-based capital of physical exercise and the holistic conception of human being in PE teachers' work]. (PhD Diss., University of Lapland, Rovaniemi, Finland).
4. Giorgi, A. (1994). A Phenomenological perspective on certain qualitative research methods. *Journal of Phenomenological Psychology, 23*, 119–135.
5. Giorgi, A. (1997). The theory, practice and evaluation of the phenomenological method as a qualitative research procedure. *Journal of Phenomenological Psychology, 28*, 235–260.
6. Perttula, J. (1995). *Kokemus psykologisena tutkimuskohteena. Johdatus fenomenologiseen psykologiaan* [Experience as a psychological research target. Introduction to phenomenological psychology].Tampere: Tampere University Press.
7. Perttula, J. (2000). Kokemuksesta tiedoksi: fenomenologisen metodin uudelleen muotoilua [From experience into knowledge: re-shaping the phenomenological method]. *Kasvatus, 31*, 428–442.
8. Fontana, A., & Frey, J. H. (2005). The interview. From Neutral stance to political involvement. In N. Denzin & Y. Lincoln (Eds.), *The Sage handbook of qualitative research* (pp. 695-727). Thousand Oaks, CA: Sage.
9. Lehtomaa, M. (2008). Fenomenologinen kokemuksen tutkimus: Haastattelu, analyysi ja ymmärtäminen [Phenomenological research on experiences: interview, analysis, and understanding]. In J. Perttula & T. Latomaa (Eds.), *Kokemuksen tutkimus: merkitys-tulkinta-*

60

ymmärtäminen [Research on experience: Meaning-interpretation-understanding] (pp. 163-197). Tampere: Juvenes Print.

10.   Magill, R. A. (2007). *Motor learning and control: Concepts and applications.* New York, NY: Mc Graw-Hill.

11.   Schmidt, R. A., & Lee, T. D. (2005). *Motor learning and performance. A behavioral emphasis.* Champaign, IL: Human Kinetics.

12.   Adams, J. A. (1971). A closed-loop theory of motor learning. *Journal of Motor Behavior, 16,* 111–150.

13.   Fitts, P. M., & Posner, M. I. (1967). *Human performance.* Belmont, CA: Brooks/Cole.

14.   Gentile, A. M. (1972). A working model of skill acquisition with application to teaching. *Quest, 17,* 3–23.

15.   Jaakkola, T. (2010). *Liikuntataitojen oppiminen ja taitoharjoittelu* [The learning of physical exercising skills and skill practicing]. Juva: PS-kustannus.

16.   Schmidt, R. A. (1975). A schema theory of discrete motor learning theory. *Psychological Review, 82,* 225–260.

17.   Vereijken, B., Whiting, H. T. A., & Beek, W. J. (1992). A dynamical systems approach to skill acquisition. *Quarterly Journal of Experimental Psychology, 45A,* 323–344.

18.   Gallahue, D. L., & Ozmun, F. C. (2006). *Understanding motor development: Infants, children, adolescents, adults.* Madison, WI: Brown and Benchmark.

19.   Trost, S. G. (2006). Public health and physical education. In D. Kirk, D. MacDonald & M. O'Sullivan (Eds.), *The handbook of physical education* (pp. 163-187). London: Sage.

20.   Aggestedt, B., & Tebelius, U. (1977). *Barns upplevelser av idrott* [Children's experiences of sport]. (PhD Thesis, University of Göteborg, Sweden].

21.   Carlson, T. (1995). We hate gym: Student alienation from physical education. *Journal of Teaching in Physical Education, 14,* 467–477.

22.   Growes, S., & Laws, C. (2000). Children's experience of physical education. *European Journal of Physical Education, 5,* 22–27.

23.   Huisman, T. (2004). *Liikunnan arviointi peruskoulussa. Yhdeksäsluokkalaisten kunto, liikuntaaktiivisuus ja koululiikuntaan asennoituminen* [PE grading at comprehensive school. Ninth-graders physical shape, activiy, and attitude toward PE]. Helsinki: Finnish National Board of Education.

24.   Gallahue, D. L., & Donelly, F. C. (2003). *Developmental physical education for all children.* Champaign, IL: Human Kinetics.

25.   Allison, P., Pissanos. B., & Sakola, S. (1990). Physical education revisited. The institutional biographies of preservice classroom teachers. *Journal of Physical Education, Recreation and Dance, 61*(5), 76–79.

26.   Deci, E. L., & Ryan, R. M. (2000). The "what" and "why" of goal pursuits: Human needs and the selfdetermination of behavior. *Psychological Inquiry, 11,* 227–268.

27.   Liukkonen, J., Jaakkola, T., & Soini, M. (2007). Motivaatioilmasto liikunnano-petuksessa [Motivational climate in PE]. In P. Heikinaro-Johansson & T. Huovinen (Eds.), *Näkökulmia liikuntapedagogiikkaan* [Perspectives in PE-pedagogy]. Helsinki: WSOY.

28.   Soini, M. (2006). *Motivaatioilmaston yhteys yhdeksäsluokkakaisten fyysiseen aktiivisuuteen ja viihtymiseen koulun liikuntatunneilla* [The connection between motivational atmosphere with ninthgraders' physical activity and contentment in PElessons]. Jyväskylä: University of Jyväskylä

29.   O'Rand, A. (2006). Stratification and the life course. The Forms of life-course capital and their interrelationships. In R. Binstock & L. George (Eds.), *Handbook of aging and the social sciences* (pp. 145-162). San Diego, CA: Academic Press.

30.   Karisto, A., & Konttinen, R. (2004). *Kotiruokaa, kotikatua, kaukomatkailua. Tutkimus ikääntyvien elämäntyyleistä* [Home meal, soap operas, far-off traveling. Research on the life-styles of the elderly]. Helsinki: Palmenia-kustannus.

31.   Hyry-Honka, O. (2008). *Terveyspääoma kouluyhteisössä seitsemäsluokkalaisten käsitysten valossa* [Health capital at school in the light of seventhgraders' opinions]. (PhD Diss., University of Lapland, Rovaniemi, Finland.)

32.   Bourdieu, P. (1996). The forms of capital. In J. G. Richardson (Ed.), *Handbook of theory and research for the sociology of education* (pp. 241-258). New York, NK: Greenwood Press.

33.   Bourdieu, P. (1990). Structures, habitus, practices. In P. Bourdieu (Ed.), *The logic of practice* (pp. 52-65). Cambridge: Polity.

34.   Bourdieu, P. (1977). *Outline of theory of practice.* Cambridge: Cambridge University Press.

35.   DeFrance, J. (1995). The anthropological sociology of Pierre Bourdieu: Genesis, concepts, relevance. *Sociology of Sport Journal, 12*, 121–131.

36.   Bourdieu, P. (1978). Sport and social class. *Social Science Information, 17*(6), 819–840.

37.   Shilling, C. (1991). Educating the body: physical capital and the production of social inequalities. *Sociology, 25*(4), 653–672.

38.   Shilling, C. (2004). Physical capital and situated action: a new direction for corporeal sociology. *British Journal of Sociology of Education, 25*(4), 473–487.

39.   Roos, J. P. (1987). Pelin säännöt: intellektuellit, luokat ja kieli [The rules of the game: intellectuels, classes, and language]. In P. Bourdieu (Ed.), *Sosiologian kysymyksiä* [Questions of sociology] (pp. 7-28). Jyväskylä: Gummerus.

40.   Bourdieu, P. (1984). *Distinction. A social critique of the judgement of taste.* Cambridge: Harvard University Press.

41.   Dumais, S. (2002). Cultural capital, gender and school success: The role of habitus. *Sociology of Education, 75*(1), 44–68.

42.   Stempel, C. (2005). Adults' participation sports as cultural capital: A Test of Bourdieu's theory of the field of sport. *International Review for the Sociology of Sport, 40*, 411–432.

43.   Mehus, I. (2005). Distinction through sport consumption: Spectators of soccer, basketball, and ski-jumping. *International Review for the Sociology of Sport, 40*(3), 321–333.

44.   Thrane, C. (2001). Sport spectatorship in Scandinavia: A class phenomenon? *International Review for the Sociology of Sport, 36*(2), 149–163.

45.   Wilson, T. C. (2002). The Paradox of social class and sports involvement: The Roles of cultural and economical capital. *International Review for the Sociology of Sport, 37*(1), 5–16.

46.   Light, R. (2001). *The body in the social world and the social world in the body: Applying Bourdieu's work to analyses of physical activity in schools.* http://www.aare.edu.au/01pap/lig01450.htm.

47.   Välipakka, I. (2005). Liikkuminen ja kehollisen eläytymisen taito: Fyysinen pääoma sosiaalisessa toimijuudessa [The ability of physical exercise and bodily empathizing. Physical capital in social actorship]. *Niin & Näin, 45*(2), 57–63.

48.   Klemola, T. (1995). *Liikunta tienä kohti varsinaista itseä. Liikunnan projektien fenomenologinen tarkastelu* [Physical exercise as a way toward the actual self. A phenomenological study on physical exercising projects]. Tampere: FITTY.

49.   Kunnari, A. (2006). *Liikunnalliset oppimiskokemukset liikunnanopettajiksi opiskelevien ihmiskäsityksenja liikuntapääoman muovaajina* [Sportive learning and teaching experiences as shaping PE-teacher students' ideas of man and capital of physical exercise]. (Unpublished Licentiate Thesis, University of Lapland, Rovaniemi, Finland.)

62

50.   Husserl, E. (1995). *Fenomenologian idea. Viisi luentoa* [The idea of phenomenology. Five lectures]. Helsinki: Loki-Kirjat.
51.   Hjerppe, R. (1997). Sosiaalinen pääoma – tutkimisen arvioinen käsite [Social capital – a concept worth researching]. *Hyvinvointikatsaus, 1*(97), 26–29.
52.   Zacheus, T. (2009). Liikunnan merkitykset vuosina 1923-1988 syntyneiden suomalaisten nuoruudessa [The meanings of physical exercise in Finnish people's youth who were born in 1923-1988]. *Liikunta & Tiede, 46*(6), 34–40.
53.   Koski, P., & Tähtinen, J. (2005). Liikunnan merkitykset nuoruudessa [The meanings of physical exercising in youth]. *Nuorisotutkimus, 23*(1), 3–21.
54.   Lehmuskallio, M. (2008). Kulttuuriset merkitykset lasten ja nuorten liikuntakulutuksen taustalla [Cultural meanings in children's and youngsters' sport activity]. *Liikunta & Tiede, 45*(4), 20–23.
55.   Eichberg, H. (1987). *Liikuntaa harjoittavat ruumiit* [Exercising bodies]. Tampere: Vastapaino.
56.   Honkonen, R., & Suoranta, J. (1999). Junioriurheilun monet totuudet [The many truths of junior sports]. In R. Honkonen & J. Suoranta (Eds.), *Höntsyä vai tehovalmennusta? Kirjoituksia joukkueurheilun junioritoiminnasta* [Easy-going or crash-training? Writings about the junior activity of team sport]. Tampere: TAJU.
57.   Renson, R. (1991). Homo Movens: In Search of paradigms for the study of humans in movement. In R. J. Park & H. M. Eckert (Eds.), *New possibilities, new paradigms?* (pp. 100-114). Champaign, IL: American Academy of Physical Education Papers.
58.   Taks, M., Renson, R., & Vanreusel, B. (1999). Organised sport in transition: Development, structure and trends of sports clubs in Belgium. In K. Heinemann (Ed.), *Sport clubs in various European countries* (pp. 183–223). Schorndorf: Hofmann.

The Fourth Level of Health Literacy

Maija Rask, Satu Uusiautti and Kaarina Määttä

The World Health Organization defines health literacy as cognitive and social skills that determine individuals' motivation and ability to receive, understand, and use information in a way that promotes and maintains people's health[1]. Scott Simonds was the first to define the concept of health literacy in 1974 in Health Education Monograph[2, see 3]. Students should be provided as good literacy in health issues as they do in other traditional school subjects. Because insufficient health education is the reason for poor health literacy, all school levels should provide at least the minimum of health education. However, health literacy is not considered a natural part of the education system[3]. The Jakarta Declaration[4] notes the strengthening of health literacy as one of the health promotion strategies[5].

The international discussion over health literacy often leans on the levels of health literacy created by Don Nutbeam[6]: basic/functional health literacy, communicative/interactive health literacy, and critical health literacy[see also 7,8,9]. The lowest level of health literacy means that people know about health risks and health services. Health education encourages people to participate in health programs, vaccination programs, and screenings. Traditional health education and health education data function as the means. In addition, information is passed through people's networks and contacts, and the media. The approach does not aim at personal contacts or independency[6,10]. The basic health literacy consists of the fundamentals of hygiene, nutrition, security, drugs, human relationships, parenthood, and sexuality[6].

The goal of communicative health literacy is an individual with the ability to function independently, increased motivation, and self-confidence. Action aims at benefitting the individual human being. The societal benefits come from the influence on social norms and increased group activity. Health education is tailored to meet special needs[6,11]. The level of communicative health literacy evinces the late-20th-century pursuit of improving people's health skills and developing environments that support individual people. For example, health education programs aimed at increasing personal and social skills and behavioral changes make a good example of the development of communicative health literacy[6].

Critical health literacy aims at personal and communal empowerment. It strengthens people's persistency in times of facing social and economic trouble. People with critical health literacy can change general and organizational practices related to health, and communicate with leaders and politicians to realize changes they consider important[see also 11]. Health education that aims at critical health literacy focuses merely on the promotion of the health of the population instead of individuals[6]. Health literacy that is acquired early in life affects health positively during the whole life span[12].

Tones[3] criticizes that the concept of health literacy has expanded faraway from its original meaning. The new concept makes the ambiguous health promotion concepts even more confusing. It has almost become a synonym for empowerment which is a central principle of health promotion action. Kickbusch[13] considered it necessary to distinguish health literacy and health promotion from mostly Freirean viewpoint of empowerment and the survival of American weak health literacy within the healthcare system. However, Kickbusch[8] defends the division of health literacy into three because it offers a way of discussing health promotion. Canadian researchers have suggested that health literacy could be expanded to cover also social, cultural, and environmental dimensions[14].

Christina Zarcadoolas et al.[15] expanded the definition of health literacy after the threat of bioterrorism in the United States in 2001. Their model is divided into basic, cultural, scientific, and civic health literacy. In this definition, basic health literacy covers reading, talking, writing, and interpretation of numbers. Cultural health literacy refers to the ability to recognize collective beliefs, habits, ideologies, and social identities when interpreting health-related information. Scientific health literacy includes knowledge about the basic scientific concepts, ability to understand technical entities, uncertainty of science, and fast changes. Civic health literacy covers media literacy, and awareness of civic and societal processes and the influence of individual health-related decision on national health. Zarcadoolas et al.[15] support the wide ethical and political viewpoint of seeing health as the resource of life mentioned in Ottawa Charter for Health Promotion.

Brey et al.[16] define health literacy as the ability to search, interpret, and understand basic information about health and use the information to promote health. They divide health literacy into four parts: A critical thinker studies the health problem and creates a solution. A responsible citizen considers that he or she has the responsibility to maintain the community healthy, safe, and free from fear. A life-long learner recognizes the need to use information about health during his or her whole life. An efficient communicator expresses beliefs, ideas, and information about health.

The unestablished nature of the concept of health literacy can be seen in the diverging names of the levels of literacy[7,6,17]. In this research, the first level of health literacy is considered the basic health literacy. Likewise, the ambiguity of the concept is seen in the emergence of new expressions such as media literacy[18], medical health literacy[9], and media health literacy[19]. The levels of media health literacy are the ability to identify health information, recognize the influence of information on health behavior, analyze critically information, and express intentions to act. These levels seems to somewhat correspond to the levels of health literacy developed by Nutbeam.

Ferguson[20] studied mothers' health literacy as it affects both children's and the generational health. Peerson and Saunders[9] mention that health literacy is studied from many points of view. Mancuso[1] recognizes the connection between health literacy and education, library science, healthcare, national health, and mental health. The educational context forms the original starting point for discussing health literacy. Environment, culture, purposes of information, language, learning together, and sharing describe the educational connections of health literacy. Mancuso points out the need for further analyses of health literacy.

Research shows that people with limited health literacy have high costs of medical treatments [e.g.,1], and they frequently use healthcare services instead of preventive health services. They are not interested in health news and do not really understand the treatment of chronic illnesses. Thus, their behavior threatens health[21]. This is why health literacy studies started mostly in hospitals starting from the 21st century because it was important from the point of view of prevention of illnesses and health promotion[22, see also 7].

Measurements of health literacy were developed after finding out in 1992 literacy research that over 10% of Americans, which means about 40-44 million people, had very poor literacy[22,23,24,25,26,27,28]. Mostly the measurement of health literacy has focused on the evaluation of basic health literacy[7]. Wu et al.[30] also remind of the lack of tools to measure youngsters' health literacy[see also 18,31].

TOFHLA (The Test of Functional Health Literacy) is a test that measures basic health literacy in adults, while health literacy among Spanish-speaking people is measured by TOFHLA-S. The testing takes about 22 minutes. It measures reading comprehension and numeric understanding. TOFHLA test is regarded as a reliable way of testing patients' ability to understand the health information they receive[24]. Later on, a S-TOFHLA measurement taking only 12 minutes had been developed. This was used for measuring health literacy among Taiwanese youth[12]. TOFHLA measures also have predicted patients' health improvement[22,32,33,34,35]. REALM (the Rapid Estimate of Adult Literacy in Medicine) is a test aimed for adults. It includes 66 words related to health and medicine that become more difficult gradually[22,32]. Among others, Lincoln et al.[29] have used this test when studying the connection between American substance abusers' low health literacy and depression symptoms[see also 36].

To measure health literacy, a new quick test in English and in Spanish was developed for the use of primary healthcare. This Newest Vital Sign (NVS) test includes six questions about nutrition. The test takes 3 minutes[37]. The new Health Activities Literacy Scale (HALS) is not so illness-centered than the previous ones. It includes a written and quantitative section and documentary data about health promotion, health protection, prevention of diseases, healthcare, and healthcare systems[10,38]. In addition, Mancuso[35] mentions the Medical Achievement Reading Test (MART) and the Short Assessment of Health Literacy for Spanish Speaking

66

Adults (SALSHA). The Wide Range Achievement Test (WRAT) is also very popular test measuring limited health literacy[39]. Qualitative measures of health literacy have not been as popular as quantitative ones[19,40,41]. However, it is important to measure citizens' health literacy because researchers have noted that low health literacy often leads to big societal costs[see also 42].The purpose of this study is to analyze how health literacy appears in the light of general upper secondary education students' test answers in health education. Based on the results, the levels of health literacy were re-evaluated and the possibilities of developing the school subject of health education were discussed. The fundamental contribution is to point out the relevance of health education in how the youth reach the highest levels of health literacy.

Method

Background of the Study

Health education became an independent subject in basic education, and in general and vocational upper secondary education in Finland. In the spring 2007, the first test in health education as a part of the Finnish Matriculation Examination for general upper secondary education students was held. In the curriculum for general upper secondary education, health education is defined in the following manner:

> Health education is a school subject based on multidisciplinary knowledge and its purpose is to promote skills that support health, well-being, and safety. This knowledge in manifested as intellectual, social, functional, and ethical abilities and skills of emotional regulation and information acquisition. Health literacy includes the readiness to be responsible for the promotion of one's own and others' health. In health education of general upper secondary education, health and maladies and health promotion and illness prevention and treatment are considered from the points of view of the individual, family, community, and society.[43, p. 210.]

The matriculation examination in health education measures students' ability to define the core concepts of the subjects correctly and precisely. Especially, students' maturity becomes evident in how they write about their knowledge and understanding, and how they structure their test answers and arguments. The purpose of this study is to discuss the following question: How does health literacy appear in the light of general upper secondary education students' test answers in health education?

The Data

The research data consisted of 611 essays that were the test answers in health education—486 essays from the examination held in spring 2007 and 125 essays from the examination held in fall 2007. The essays covered altogether eight questions about health education. Eighty-one candidates for the spring 2007 matriculation examination and 60 candidates for the fall 2007 matriculation examination participated in this research; altogether 141 candidates—37 of them were men and 104 were women. The participants were aged between 18 and 20 years. All candidates were Finnish speaking.

The test in health education includes ten questions, and students can answer to six of them. Five test questions from the spring 2007 matriculation examination were selected for this study, the data were complemented by three questions from the fall 2007 examination.

Test answers were transcribed and altogether they comprise 374 pages. The research was phenomenological-hermeneutical, in which a human being is seen as a researcher and research participant[44,45,46]. The hermeneutic research method tries to understand and interpret the life world[45,47,48,49]. The data were analyzed through qualitative content analysis. Deduction was employed when drawing conclusions[45]. During the analysis, scattered data were put together and condensed carefully without losing any essential information[50]. The analysis leaned on the levels of health literacy and Bloom's taxonomy as well as on the learning objectives of the national core curriculum for health education in general upper secondary education. Candidates' answers in Matriculation Examination represent natural research data because they exist regardless of the research and thus participants were not influenced by the researcher or the research setting. In the data excerpts included in this article, the letter "F" refers to a female candidate and the letter "M" refers to a male candidate. The numbers illustrate the candidates' serial number in the data: numbers 1–81 refer to spring candidates and 82–141 fall candidates.

The hierarchical definition of health literacy was selected as a suitable basis for the study as it illustrates increasing knowledge, too[6,11]. The levels of health literacy were operationalized according to Nutbeam's and St Leger's descriptions. Each task selected for the study was separately categorized into the different levels of health literacy. Abductive analysis was applied in this study. In addition, the categorization was consulted by Bloom's taxonomy: the six levels start from remembering advancing all the way through understanding, applying, analyzing, making synthesis, and finally to evaluating and creating new[51,52,53]. Learning objectives for health education were studied side-by-side when analyzing the test answers. The learning objectives were also categorized according to the levels of health literacy. Categorizing the answers was challenging because they did not always represent just one level but many. Therefore, it is possible that they could be categorized differently. If an answer seemed to represent two levels, it was categorized into the upper level of health literacy.

Results

The students' answers were evaluated as the basic-level health literacy when they remembered and were capable of describing the issues asked in the question. These answers had no or little reasoning. The curriculum for general upper secondary education includes basically the goals of basic health literacy, namely students are expected to know national diseases and national health and be familiar with the prevention of the most common infectious and national diseases and their treatments[43]. According to Bloom's taxonomy, the student can recognize the phenomenon and remembers and can describe factors related to it. Test answers that represented basic health literacy covered approximately 23% of all answers (n = 140).

Communicative health literacy consisted of test answers in which the students wrote about the significance of the way of life to health, mentioned motivation to pursue healthy life and familiarize with health information. Of 611 test answers, 229 represented communicative health literacy, which equals 37% of all answers.

Those answers that fulfilled the criteria of basic and communicative health literacy and in which students wrote about the wish to work for the communal health and its promotion were categorized as critical health literacy; 194 test answers (32%) belonged to this category. In addition, 48 test answers (8%) did not meet the criteria of any level of health literacy. The reason was either too brief an answer or digressing from the subject.

A New Level of Health Literacy: Holistic Health Literacy

As the analysis proceeded, it became clear that the three aforementioned levels of health literacy were not enough for describing the depth of students' test answers in the health education test. The fourth level was created which was called the highest level of health literacy. This level is called holistic health literacy. The concept of holistic health literacy was also introduced in the youth research project among indigenous people in Canada[14].

The abundant and versatile empirical data gave reason to create this new level after many phases of analysis. Poskiparta[54] has stated that a person who promotes his or her health acts in a way that increases the societal value of health. According to Jakonen[55], the parts of holistic health are physical, mental, social, sexual, spiritual, and emotional-life health. All these factors are influenced by societal, cultural, and physical environment. Societal health emerges from the interaction between a human being and his or her socio-cultural environment.

The concept of health literacy has been criticized in the Finnish health discussion. Hoikkala and Hakkarainen[56] have demanded a societal perspective on theoretical and empirical research on health literacy. Puuronen[57] considers emphasis on the cognitive side of health as the weakness of the concept of health literacy.

Health literacy is not only built on cognitive construction of health-related information but it also includes the understanding of one's own and others' well-being. Also Jakonen[55] has encouraged criticizing the use of the concept. Jakonen asks whether the concept of health literacy increases the value of individual and communal health promotion or whether it lacks practical application value.

Jakarta Declaration includes socio-policy, healthy environment, improvement of communal action, development of personal skills, and renewal of health services as parts of efficient health promotion[4]. This declaration convinces that the three levels of health literacy might not be enough. Based on the test answers in health education test, holistic health literacy consists of the following dimensions:
1. tolerance;
2. understanding the culture as wide and multidimensional phenomenon;
3. environmental consciousness; and
4. analyzing the state of the world from various points of view.

All these dimensions include argumentation and deep contemplation from a wider perspective than just regarding one's own healthcare. These societally relevant dimensions of health could be found in the students' test answers.

Tolerance

Tolerance was strongly emphasized in some test answers. Students highlighted how important it is to accept dissimilarity. They listed different people groups such as the overweight, immigrants, unemployed, poor, Romany, black, elderly, and even the youth who differ from the mass. "A human being is a social creature who needs acceptance," wrote one female student (N99).

Everyone has to be treated well regardless of their background. "Also immigrants are entitled to equal and humane treatment in Finland" (N8). Answers that manifested holistic health literacy showed everyday realism and compassion.

> Especially immigrants and other minorities have often a difficult situation. They do not have such a large network around them supporting them like the majority of the Finnish people do. They often get less support from their immediate neighborhood and the society. Racism and discrimination but also legal actions such as admittance of citizenship create more difficult circumstances in order to have a balanced, satisfactory, and healthy life. (N34)

The basis of the pedagogical ethos of health education is to learn how to confront various people and behave naturally. The purpose is to increase students' sensitivity toward health which includes tolerance and ability to accept differences in health. Sensitivity also means appreciation of health and respect for the maintenance of health[58].

Understanding of Culture as a Wide and Multidimensional Phenomenon

Holistic health literacy means that one perceives health more than just absence of diseases.

> The health-related differences between various population groups can be explained by the attitudes and habits of groups and their general attitude to life. Those groups who are more positive on average and who have more social support are usually healthier than others. (N18)

Zarcadoolas et al.[15] point out that cultural literacy includes the ability to recognize and use common collective beliefs, habits, worldviews, and social identities. Health-related information has to be considered consisting of cultural understanding, science, and individual and collective actions[14].

Likewise, answers representing holistic health literacy showed that the student realized how cultural differences affect people's health. One female student (N10) pointed out this by saying that "health is not distributed equally. It is affected by our opportunities that are based on our heredity and environment but also by our orientation." These types of answers also showed awareness of health cultures across the world and ability to compare cultures.

> Differences in health are huge. The biggest difference is between the rich and poor countries in which life expectancy can differ over 30 years from each other. This concerns also the European Union, especially after getting the new member states from the Eastern Europe. The Finns have pure drinking water and only a few are poor when compared to incomes in developing countries. (N42)

Understanding of health culture also requires knowledge of history and development. The following quotation illustrates how a male student contemplated the reasons for increasing depression among the youth. Traditions and culture lay the foundation for communality, which affects social well-being.

> The worlds, habits, manners, and norms change. Today is different from the time 30, 50, or hundred years ago. It is difficult to think that typical melancholia would have increased along the course of time. This is why it would be necessary to focus more on analyzing the role of the environment in youth's depression. (M34)

A female student (N33) wrote that "men consider going to doctor as a sign of weakness whereas women as taking care of themselves." A male student (M22) had pointed out that "ideal women and men are far from an average person." Traditional differences in men's and women's roles affect people's well-being and quality of life. "Our culture sets different demands, behavioral norms, and goals for women and men. Men are still expected to support the family" (N20).

In this study, students considered unhealthy life style and busy rhythm of life and environmental degradation as the most significant health threats. In Aarva and Pasanen's [59] study, men named unhealthy life style was the biggest danger while women thought that environmental degradation and busy life style were the most serious factors threatening health. The researchers concluded that men were more likely to emphasize traditional issues in life style but women perceived also the importance of peace of mind and environmental protection for health [59].

The general upper secondary education students saw culture as a factor that promotes health. They mentioned libraries, different kinds of schools, and churches that offer opportunities to study and maintain mental vitality. Cultural hobbies together with sportive hobbies and social contacts that are formed along these support mental and physical well-being which leads to better health in general. Hyyppä [60] has stated that cultural activity d rectly affects people's well-being; likewise, cultural acts and hobbies promote health.

"If one wants to be as healthy as possible, one should be a Finland-Swedish young woman who lives in a middle-size municipality near good services but also near to the nature," wrote a female student (N41) in a sarcastic style. Many test answers showed understanding of the social capital as a factor that promotes health. "In addition to healthy life style and good livelihood, the Finland-Swedes have a wide social network promoting mental, physical, and, of course, social health. They get support for each other, work together for a common goal" (N49). According to Aarva and Pasanen[59], this kind of positive attitude toward life is regarded as a health-promoting factor.

Environmental Consciousness

Test answers that represented holistic health literacy showed environmental consciousness and the importance of the state of the environment to health. Environmental consciousness was expressed, for example, as concern over methods of food production, sufficiency of food, and unequal distribution of food in the world. The method of food production can be bad for the environment. "Even the food production has increased so tremendously in the world that it is impossible to produce enough food supplies without consumption and eroding the nature. Likewise, infectious diseases among the livestock are dangers of today" (N74). Sufficiency and availability of food concerned many students, too:

> The world has about three kilos of food for everyone per day. But as it is unevenly distributed, there is abundance and overweight in some parts and famine and malnutrition in other parts. Especially, fatness is a problem in industrialized and rich countries, such as Finland. (N81)

Georg Henrik von Wright[61] analyzed how the world population has increased fast because of the high living standards but which has led to the destruction of nature, exhaustion of natural resources, and narrower areas of cultivable land. The answers also included discussion of domestic production of food supplies and the healthiness of food in the light of environmental questions. Domestic food production and functional health products were considered health promoting. Local food was seen as a good option.

> Finnish people should favor local, domestic vegetables, breads, and meats. This way we could support domestic economy, sustainable development with lower carbon dioxide emissions and decreased the dominance of supranational companies in the food market. (N79)

The students' test answers also showed the different habits of people living in cities and in the countryside. The latter group can eat more organic products and do not suffer from pollution as much as the city people do. Students also wrote much about fatness because one task asked them to discuss fatness. While it was often discussed in a relatively tolerant tone, it was sometimes disapproved too. "Getting fatter is against sustainable development. Nor is an over-weight person interested in the original country of their wood or food supplies, not to mention the contents of the food" (N79).

Answers also included a sort of gratitude of having been born in Finland and wish that people would see the meaning of it. "The Finnish people have to learn how to respect themselves, health, and environment so that they would see the holistic influence of their choices" (N14). In Aarva and Pasanen's[59] study, especially the youth considered their own life style a bigger health risk than the pollution of the nature. Environmental issues were at the top of the citizens' priorities. However, according to Helve[62], many youngsters would be ready to compromise their living standards for the nature protection or underprivileged.

The State of the World and Criticism toward Western Countries

Holistic health literacy also shows concern over the state of the world. Students' answers representing this level of health literacy included comparisons of the modern western life style with the situation in developing countries. The evaluations not only disapproved over-consumption and constant busyness but also expressed the demand on moderation.

Students pointed out that many of the problems in developed countries were connected to nutrition. The problem is difficult to solve because it is such a personal matter. The following quotation highlights the core of the problem: "Western societies idolizes thinness and fatness is regarded as disgusting. However, fatness is one of the most common causes of death in western countries" (N78).

Students' answers also brought out the influence of family. Reasons for too little sleep could be found already from childhood: "Parents have started to be less disciplinarian and having a computer or TV in a child's own room affect the control over the time the child sleeps." Physical exercising was mentioned often and voluntariness was emphasized in many answers.

Students also criticized the commercialism of the modern life. Because the test had a food advertisement as an example, students criticized mostly advertising of food supplies. "The purpose of stores is not to promote people's health but marketing and making money" (N35). The answers understood the storekeeper's point of view, too. People cannot just blame advertising and storekeepers for their own gourmandize and weight-gaining. "Storekeeping is a profession and they want to earn their keep. . . . At least, according to the modern conception, the consumer has the responsibility for knowing the healthiness of the food supplies they buy" (N59).

Students who had reached the level of holistic health literacy appeared humanitarian. This could be interpreted from their ways of writing about inequality between people and in opportunities in life across the world. Poverty was mentioned as the world's deadliest disease. "When considered from a world-wide perspective, it is unfair that some people have energy more than they need while some die from hunger" (N73). Students also perceived that poverty is not just the problem of developing countries.

> For example, millions of people in the United States of America living on the margins of poverty, and they can afford only the cheap fast food. So, even if they had knowledge about healthy food, money hinders them from buying it. American schools also offer fast food and corridors have soda and candy vending machines. (N44)

Discussion of the Concept of Holistic Health Literacy

The dimensions of holistic health literacy are tolerance, cultural and environmental awareness, and interest in the state of the world (see Figure 1). This level of health literacy was reached by students who could be called humanitarian. In addition, philanthropy and altruism seem to be related to holistic health literacy. In addition to these, the cognitive aspect of social responsibility leads to docility[63].

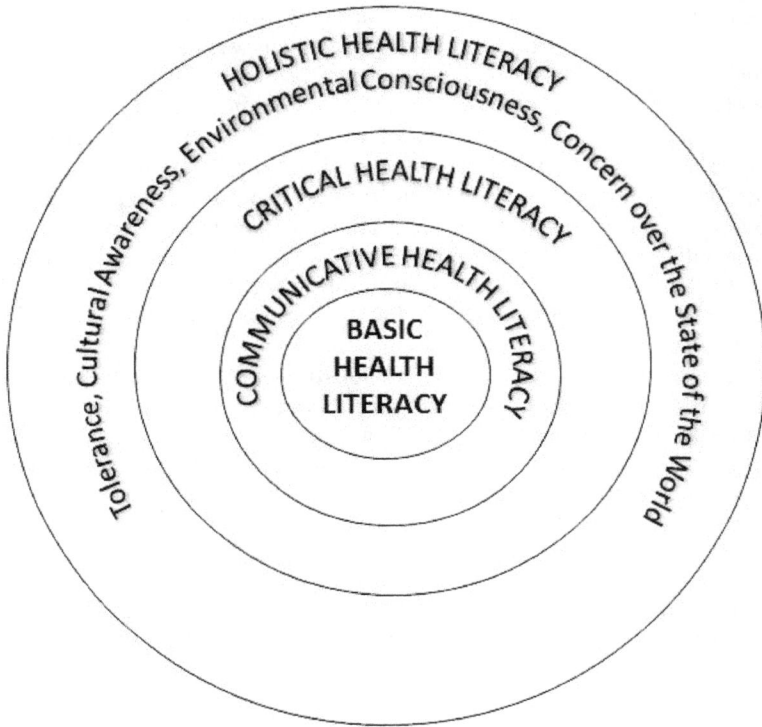

Figure 1. The four levels of health literacy

When the level of holistic health literacy is compared to Osler and Starkey's[64] research on cosmopolitan citizenship, they seem to have plenty in common. Educating students as cosmopolitans aims at teaching how to distinguish and see the connection between national and global society. This means a holistic approach in education. Cosmopolitanism means solidarity and humanist attitude to other people. It also means willingness to solve future problems in cooperation. Osler and Starkey[64] suggest that education should pay attention to globalization and learning outside the school world. Educating students as cosmopolitan citizens also means peace education, adaptation of the duties related to human rights, and appreciation of democracy.

The idea of educating cosmopolitanism harks back to the UNESCO conference in Paris in 1995. The purpose is to raise citizens who respect peace, human rights, and democracy[65]. These objectives can also be found in the thematic entities of the curriculum for general upper secondary education. The theme of Active citizenship and enterprise seems to emphasize more enterprise and citizenship at the moment. The theme of Sustainable development includes good goals, but it is not clear how they can be met because Sustainable development is not a school subject per se. In addition, cultural identity and cultural knowledge are thematic entities having goals promoting cosmopolitanism.

People whose health literacy is holistic are tolerant and accept people's dissimilarity. Cultural awareness means that they perceive the influence of various health cultures on health and realize that art in its different forms also promotes health. Moreover, holistic health literacy means that people are environmentally conscious and concerned over the state of nature in their home countries and across the world. They perceive the connection between abundant life in Western countries and scarcity in developing countries and are willing to look for a solution. In all, the following characteristics describe people who have reached the holistic level of health literacy:

- they are tolerant to various groups of people;
- they are antiracist;
- they are widely aware of the influence of cultural differences on health;
- they are aware of the importance of art and civilization for health;
- they understand the significance of social capital for physical, mental, and social health;
- they are concerned about the environmental threats;
- they appreciate and protect environment;
- they criticize the evils of western life because they pose a threat to health; and
- they want to promote health globally.

Conclusion: How to Develop the School Subject of Health Education?

American researchers and educationalists have announced that healthy students are better students[66,67] and, in Canada, health literacy is to be included in curricula from basic education to adult education[68]. The aims must be high and the development of holistic health literacy among the youth would be easier if the subject of health education was developed in the direction that supports the emergence of characteristics listed in the previous chapter. In Finland, the current curriculum provides a good basis for such health education. The subject has already existed 10 years and it has developed a lot. Teacher education in the subject has been established. In addition, there are plenty of text books available, and the Internet also has appropriate learning materials. The Finnish National Board of Education provides a teachers' internet service and offers an electric health library for the use of teachers and students[69]. General upper secondary education students' knowledge and skills in maintaining their own health and ability to discuss health-related social issues have improved considerably in a short time[70].

Based on the research results, the targets of development in health education can be divided into three groups. The most important measure would be to increase time allocation so that health education could meet the objectives written in the curriculum. The ideas and contents of the subject are so wide and profound that learning and teaching them requires time.

Second, the subject should become popular also among boys. We know that the better education one has, the better is his or her health also[71,72,73]. Nowadays, men form the minority of general upper secondary education graduates in Finland. In 2007, there were 33,000 graduates and less than 14,000 of them were men. In the same year, health education was selected in the test by 6,625 graduates of whom only 1,472 were men. Women scored better in the health education test than men[74]. In this study, gender was not the basis of selecting test answers: 37 were men and 104 women, and even in this sample, women performed better.

Another reason for getting men interested in the subject of health education is that many national diseases come from an unhealthy life style. In this study, students discussed differences between women and men. Women want to look good and maintain their health while men go to a doctor only when that is the last option. The Finnish men's way of taking care of health does not follow healthy life style[75].

One way of making health education more interesting to boys is to use more student-centered teaching methods[55]. According to research, men are interested in physical exercising, fitness tests, and muscles[59], and dating and sex education[76]. All these can be discussed in health education. Furthermore, Koski[77] points out that since men and women perceive health differently, health education could have genderspecific entities. Likewise, general upper secondary education could collaborate with other important institutions such as the army[78] and sport clubs [77].

Third, health education has to constantly be updated. It means that values and human life could be widely discussed in health education. The hectic modern life was questioned in this study too. How to pay attention to inactivity, stillness, and spirituality[59] in health education? Would it be possible to include a moment of rest in health education lessons [57,see also 79]?

Aarva and Pasanen's[59] and Pihlström's[79] wishes correspond to Kannas's description of the nature of health education. Health education is a subject that requires ability to discuss values. The ethos of health education resembles philosophy as it aims at wondering, criticizing, asking, developing thinking skills, and reasoning. Reflecting values and appreciations on one's own health, diseases, risks, and even death necessitate contemplation and ethical tools.

Aarva and Pasanen's[59], Pihlström's[79], and Kannas's[58] findings support the need for increasing lessons in health education. Discussing the difficult issues requires time, and health education as a subject could promote the more peaceful life style. In addition, many students thought that fear of the future is one of the reasons for increasing depression in the youth. Health education as a subject could help youngsters at the time they form their identity.

Because students are worried about the state of the world and environment, these issues should be discussed in health education lessons, too. The youth seem to adopt an ecological world view and change their habits while they criticize the society and politics[62].

Keeping the subject updated means that health education has to pay more attention to environmental awareness. In the values of general upper secondary education, this is clearly mentioned: "General upper secondary education has to emphasize the principles of sustainable development and provide means of facing the challenges of the changing worlds." The development of health education needs to follow these principles as well[43]. Of the thematic entities, Sustainable development, increases environmental awareness the best. Although thematic entities in general upper secondary education are cross-curricular and can unify teaching, they are not paid enough attention in education. Some of the objectives of sustainable development could be chosen as the objectives of health education, such as: "The student knows how to co-operate for the better future locally, nationally, and globally" and "The student discusses sustainable life style, production and society that are nature-preserving and eco-efficient, community and society that strengthen their social capital, and culture that cares for the natural foundation from generation to generation."

Health-related studies have concentrated on themes around one problem at a time; while a holistic and positive approach to health has been minimal[80]. This study aimed to contribute to the discussion by introducing new perspectives on health education and citizens' health literacy. In the modern world, themes of solidarity, cosmopolitanism, and shared concern over environmental issues make a salient, downright inevitable part of health education. The foundation of people' health appreciation is laid at school; but in order to fulfill this goal, health education needs constant updating and understanding about the globalized world's requirements of people's health literacy pointed out in this study.

References

1. Mancuso, J. M. (2008). Health literacy: A concept/dimensional analysis. *Nursing and Health Science, 10*, 248-255.
2. Ratzan, S. C. (2001). Health literacy: Communication for the public good. *Health Promotion International, 16*(2), 207-214.
3. Tones, K. (2002). Health literacy: New wine in old bottles? Editorial. *Health Education Research, 17*(3), 287-290.
4. *Jakarta Declaration on Leading Health Promotion into 21st Century*. (1997). http://www.who.int.hpr/NPH/docs/jakarta_declaration_en.pdf
5. Nutbeam, D. (1998). Health promotion glossary. *Health Promotion International, 13*(4), 349-364.

78

6. Nutbeam, D. (2000). Health literacy as a public health goal: A challenge for contemporary health education and communication strategies into the 21st century. *Health Promotion International, 15*(3), 259-267.
7. Abel, T. (2008). Cultural capital and social inequality in health. *Journal of Epidemiology and Community Health, 62*(7), e13.
8. Kickbusch, I. S. (2002). Health literacy: A search for new categories. *Health Promotion International, 17*(1), 1-2.
9. Peerson, A., & Saunders, M. (2009). Health literacy revisited: What do we mean and why does it matter? *Health Promotion International, 24*(3), 285-296.
10.   Nutbeam, D. (2008). The evolving concept of health literacy. *Social Science and Medicine, 67,* 2072-2078.
11.   St Leger, L. (2001). Schools, health literacy and public health: Possibilities and challenges. *Health Promotion International, 16*(2), 197-205.
12.   Chang, L. C. (2010). Meeting the needs of diverse communities. Health literacy, selfreported status and health promoting behaviours for adolescents in Taiwan. *Journal of Clinical Nursing, 20,* 190-196.
13.   Kickbusch, I. S. (2001). Health literacy: Addressing the health and education divide. *Health Promotion International, 16,* 289-297.
14.   Stewart, S., Riecken, T., Scott, T., Tanaka, M., & Riecken, J. (2008). Expanding health literacy. Indigenous youth creating videos. *Journal of Health Psychology, 13*(2), 180-189.
15.   Zarcadoolas, C., Pleasant, A., & Greer, D. S. (2005). Understanding health literacy: An expanded model. *Health Promotion International, 20*(2), 195-203.
16.   Brey, R. A., Clark, S. E., & Wantz, M. S. (2007). Enhancing health literacy through accessing health information, products, and services: An exercise for children and adolescents. *Journal of School Health, 77*(9), 640-644.
17.   Savola, E., & Koskinen-Ollonqvist, P. (2005). *Terveyden edistäminen esimerkein. Käsitteitä ja selityksiä* [Examples of health promotion. Concepts and explanations]. Helsinki: Edita Prima.
18.   Manganello, J. A. (2008). Health literacy and adolescents: A framework and agenda for future research. *Health Education Research, 23*(5), 840-847.
19.   Levin-Zamir, D., Lemish, D., & Gofin, R. (2011). Media Health Literacy (MHL): Development and measurement of the concept among adolescents. *Health Education Research, 2*(26), 323-335.
20.   Ferguson, B. (2008). Health literacy and health disparities. The role they play in maternal and child health. *Nursing for Women's Health, 12*(4), 287-298.
21.   Wallace, L. (2006). Patients' health literacy skills: The missing demographic variable in primary care research. *Annals of Family Medicine, 4*(1), 85-86.
22.   Parker, R. (2000). Health literacy: A challenge for American patients and their care providers. *Health Promotion International, 15*(4), 277-283.
23.   Ad Hoc Committee on Health Literacy for the Council on Scientific Affairs. (1999). Health literacy: Report of the council on scientific affairs. *Journal of the American Medical Association, 281*(6), 552-557.
24.   Parker, R. M., Baker, D. W., Williams, M. V., &Nurss, J. R. (1995). The Test of Functional Health Literacy in Adults: A new instrument for measuring patients' literacy skills. *Journal of General Internal Medicine, 10,* 537-541.
25.   Carmona, R. H. (2006). Health literacy: A national priority. *Journal of General Internal Medicine, 21,* 803.
26.   Chew, L. D., Bradley, K. A., & Boyko, E. J. (2004). Brief questions to identify patients with inadequate health literacy. *Family Medicine, 36*(8), 588-594.

27.	Davis, T. C., & Wolf, M. C. (2004). Health literacy: Implications for family medicine. *Family Medicine, 36*(8), 595-598.
28.	Kripalani, S., Paashe-Orlow, M. K., Parker, R. M., & Saha, S. (2006). Advancing the field of health literacy. *Journal of General Internal Medicine, 21*, 804-805.
29.	Lincoln, A., Paashe-Orlow, M. K., Cheng, D. M., Lloyd-Travaglini, C., Caruso, C., & Saitz, R. (2006). Impact of health literacy on depressive symptoms and mental health-related quality of life among adults with addiction. *Journal of General Internal Medicine, 21*, 818-822.
30.	Wu, A. D., Begoray, D. L., MacDonald, M., Higgins, J. W., Frankish, J., & Kwan, B. (2000). Developing and evaluating a relevant and feasible instrument for measuring health literacy of Canadian high school students. *Health Promotion International, 25*(4), 444-452.
31.	Chisolm, D. J., & Buchanan, L. (2007). Measuring adolescent functional health literacy: A pilot validation of the test of functional health literacy in adults. *Journal of Adolescents Health, 41*, 312-314.
32.	Zarcadoolas, C., Pleasant, A. F., & Greer, D. (2005) Understanding health literacy: An expanded model. *Health Promotion International, 20*(2), 195-203.
33.	Gazmarian, J. A., Williams, M. V., Peel, J., Baker, & D. W. (2003). Health literacy and knowledge of chronic disease. *Patient Education & Counseling, 51*, 267–275.
34.	Jovic-Vranes, A., Bjegovic-Micanovic, V., & Marincovic, J. (2009). Functional health-literacy among primary health-care patients: Data from the Belgrade pilot study. *Journal of Public Health, 31*(4), 490-495.
35.	Mancuso, J. M. (2009). Assessment and measurement of health literacy: An integrative review on the literature. *Nursing and Health Science, 11*, 77-89.
36.	Ibrahim, S. Y., Reid, F., Shaw, A., Rowlands, G., Gomez, G. B., Chesnokov, M., et al. (2008). Validation of Health Literacy Screening Tool (REALM) in a UK population with coronary hearth disease. *Journal of Public Health, 30*(4), 449-55.
37.	Weiss, B. D., Mays, M. Z., Martz, W., Castro, K. M., DeWalt, D. A., Pignone, M. P., Mockbee, J., & Hale, F. A. (2005). Quick assessment of literacy in primary care: the newest vital sign. *Annals of Family Medicine, 3*(6), 514-22.
38.	Baker, D. W. (2006). The meaning and the measure of health literacy. *Journal of General Internal Medicine, 21*, 878-883.
39.	von Wagner, C., Steptoe, A., Wolf, M. S., & Wardle, J. (2009). Health literacy and health actions: A review and framework from health psychology. *Health Education & Behavior, 36*(5), 860-877.
40.	Adkins, N. R., & Corus, C. (2009). Health literacy for improved health outcomes: Effective capital in the marketplace. *The Journal of Consumer Affairs, 43*(2), 199-222.
41.	Ishikawa, H., Nomura, K., & Sato, M. (2008). Developing a measure of communicative and critical health literacy: A pilot study of Japanese office workers. *Health Promotion International, 23*(3), 269-275.
42.	Levy, M., & Royne, M. B. (2009). The impact of consumers' health literacy on public health. *The Journal of Consumer Affairs, 43*(2), 367-372.
43.	*Core Curriculum of General Upper Secondary Education*. (2003). Helsinki: National Board of Education.
44.	Laverty, S. M. (2003). Hermeneutic phenomenology and phenomenology: A comparison of historical and methodological considerations. *International Journal of Qualitative Methods, 2*(3), 1-29.
45.	Tuomi, J., & Sarajärvi, A. (2006). *Laadullinen tutkimus ja sisällönanalyysi* [Qualitative research and content analysis]. Jyväskylä: Gummerus.

80

46.   Zimmer, L. (2006). Methodological issues in nursing research. Qualitative meta-synthesis: A question of dialoguing with texts. *Journal of Advanced Nursing, 53*(3), 311-318.
47.   Alvesson, M., & Sköldberg, K. (1994). *Tolkning och refletion. Vetenskapsfilosofi och kvalitativ metod* [Interpretation and reflection. The philosophy of science and qualitative method]. Lund: Studentlitteratur.
48.   Anttila, P. (2005). *Ilmaisu, teos, tekeminen ja tutkiva toiminta* [Expression, product, doing, and researching]. Tallinn: AS Pakett.
49.   Gadamer, H.-G. (2009). *Hermeneutiikka. Ymmärtäminen tieteissä ja filosofiassa* [Hermeneutics. Understanding in arts and philosophy]. Tallinn: Raamatutrukikoda.
50.   Bogdan, R. C., & Biklen, S. K. (2006). *Qualitative research for education. An introduction to theory and methods.* Boston, MA: Pearson.
51.   Anderson, L. W., Krathwohl, D. R., Airasian, P. W., Cruikshank, K. A., Mayer, R. E., & Pintrich, P. R. (2001). *A taxonomy for learning, teaching, and assessing. A revision of Bloom's taxonomy of educational objectives.* Lebanon, IN: Addison Wesley Longman.
52.   Bloom, B. S. (Ed.). (1972). *Taxonomy of education objectives. Classification of educational goals.* Ann Arbor, MI: Edwards Bros.
53.   Bloom, B. S., Engelhart, M. D., Furst, E., J., Hill, W. H., & Krathwohl, D. R. (Eds.). (1956). *Taxonomy of educational objectives. The classification of educational goals.* Ann Arbor, MI: Edwards Bros.
54.   Poskiparta, M. (2002). Terveydenedistäjän ammatillisen orientoitumisen kehityskulut 1900- ja 2000-luvun Suomessa [The professional development of health promotion in the 20th and 21st century Finland]. In T. Koivisto, S. Muurinen, A. Peiponen, & E. Rajalahti (Eds.), *Hoitotyön vuosikirja 2003* [Annual of nursing 2003] (pp. 159-170). Tampere: Tammer-Paino.
55.   Jakonen, S. (2002). Terveyden lukutaito—Uusi näkökulma yksilön oman terveyden edistämiseen? [Health literacy—A new perspective on individual health promotion?] In T. Koivisto, S. Muurinen, A. Peiponen, & E. Rajalahti (Eds.), *Hoitotyön vuosikirja 2003* [Annual of nursing 2003] (pp. 121-132). Tampere: Tammer-Paino Oy.
56.   Hoikkala, T., & Hakkarainen, P. (2005). Nuorisokulttuurit terveyden lukutaitona [Youth cultures as health literacy]. In *Timantit. Terveyden edistämisen tutkimusohjelmasta* [Diamonds. On research program for health promotion] (pp. 127-141). Tampere: Juvenes Print.
57.   Puuronen, A. (2006). Mitä on terveys, tietoa, taitoa vai tajua? [What is health, knowledge, skills, or understanding?] In A. Puuronen (Ed.), *Terveystaju. Nuoret, politiikka ja käytäntö* [The health knowledge. The youth, politics, and practice] (pp. 5-19). Tampere: University of Tampere.
58.   Kannas, L. (2005). Terveystieto-oppiaineen olemusta etsimässä [Looking for the essence of health education]. In L. Kannas & H. Tyrväinen (Eds.), *Virikkeitä terveystiedon opetukseen* [Stimuli for health education] (pp. 9-18). Jyväskylä: Domus-Offset.
59.   Aarva, P., & Pasanen, M. (2005). Suomalaisten käsityksiä terveyteen vaikuttavista tekijöistä ja niissä tapahtuneita muutoksia vuodesta 1994 vuoteen 2002 [Finns' perceptions on factors related to health and changes in them from 1994 to 2002]. *Sosiaalilääketieteellinen Aikakauslehti, 42*, 57-71.
60.   Hyyppä, M. T. (2002). *Elinvoimaa yhteisöstä. Sosiaalinen pääoma ja terveys* [Vitality from the community. Social capital and health]. Keuruu: Otava.
61.   von Wright, G. H. (2001). *Hyvän muunnelmat* [Modifications of the good]. Keuruu: Otava.
62.   Helve, H. (2001). Nuorten muuttuvat arvot ja maailmankuvat [The changing values and worldviews of the youth]. In H. Helve (Ed.), *Arvot, maailmankuvat, sukupuoli* [Values, worldviews, gender] (pp. 140-172). Helsinki: Helsinki University Press.

63.   Secchi, D. (2009). The cognitive side of social responsibility. *Journal of Business Ethics, 88*, 565-581.
64.   *Declaration of the 44th Session of the International Conference on Education.* (1995). http://www.Unesco.org/education/nfsunesco/pdf/REV_74.PDF
65.   Osler, A., & Starkey, H. (2003). Learning for cosmopolitan citizenship: Theoretical debates and young people's experiences. *Educational Review, 55*(3), 243-254.
66.   Basch, C. E. (2010). *Healthier students are better learners: A missing link in school reforms to close the achievement gap.* http://www.equitycampaign.org/i/a/document/12557_EquityMastersVol6_web03082010.pdf
67.   Parker, R. M., & Kindig, D. A. (2006). Beyond the Institute of Medicine Health Literacy Report. Are the recommendations being taken seriously? *Journal of General Internal Medicine, 10*, 891-892.
68.   Rootman, I., & Gordon-El-Bihbety, D. (2008). *A vision for a health literacy Canada. Report of the expert panel on health literacy.* http://www.cpha.ca/uploads/portals/h-l/report_w.pdf
69.   Aira, T., Kannas, L., & Peltonen, H. (2008). Terveystieto [Health education]. In M. Rimpelä (Ed.), *Hyvinvoinnin ja terveyden edistäminen lukiossa. Perusraportti lukiokyselystä vuonna 2008* [The promotion of well-being and health at general upper secondary education] (pp. 50-56). Helsinki: Edita.
70.   *Finnish School Health Survey 2007, 2008, 2009, 2010.* http://info.stakes.fi/kouluterveyskysely/FI/index.htm
71.   Kantomaa, M., Tammelin, T., Ebeling, H., & Taanila, A. (2010). Liikunnan yhteys nuorten tunne-elämän ja käyttäytymisen häiriöihin, koettuun terveyteen ja koulumenestykseen [The connection between sport and emotional and behavioral disorders, perceived health, and school success in youth]. *Liikunta & Tiede, 47*(6), 30-37.
72.   Koskinen, S. (2006). Sosioekonomiset terveyserot—Suomen kansanterveyden keskeinen ongelma [Socio-economic health differences—A central problem in Finnish national health]. *Kansanterveys, 1*, 7-9.
73.   Mäkinen, T. (2011). Liikunnallinen elämäntapa—yksilön valinnasta yhteiskunnan tukemaksi mahdollisuudeksi? [Sportive life style—from an individual choice into an opportunity supported by the society?] *Liikunta & Tiede, 48*(1), 14-17.
74.   Finnish Matriculation Examination 2007. (2008). *Tilastoja ylioppilastutkinnosta* [Statistics about matriculation examination]. Vammala: Vammalan Kirjapaino.
75.   Ojanen, M. (2001). *Liiku oikein—Voi hyvin. Liikunnan merkitys hyvinvoinnille* [Exercice right—Be well. The significance of sport to well-being]. Tampere: Tammer-Paino.
76.   Cacciatore, R. (2005). Seksuaalisuus—Etu vai haitta koulutyölle? [Sexuality—An advantage or disadvantage for school work?] In H. Peltonen & L. Kannas (Eds.), *Terveystieto tutuksi—Ensiapua terveystiedon opettamiseen* [Familiarizing with health education—First aid to the teaching of health education] (pp. 147-188). Helsinki: Hakapaino.
77.   Koski, P. (2006). Merkitysten ristiaallokossa—Suhde terveyteen, alkoholiin ja liikuntaan rakentuu sosiaalisissa maailmoissa [In the riptide of meanings—The relationship with health, alcohol, and exercising is constructed in social worlds]. In A. Puuronen (Ed.), *Terveystaju. Nuoret, politiikka ja käytäntö* [Health knowledge. The youth, politics, and practice] (pp. 23-32). Tampere: University of Tampere.
78.   Ojajärvi, A. (2009). Combon kolmas ääni: Miehisen terveysmallin perinne [The third voice of combo: The tradition of masculine health model]. In T. Hoikkala, M. Salasuo, & A. Ojajärvi (Eds.), *Tunnetut sotilaat* [Known soldiers] (pp. 298-302). Jyväskylä: Gummerus.
79.   Pihlström, S. (2002). Ajattelu ja terveys: Huomioita terapeuttisesta filosofiasta ja filosofisesta terapiasta [Thinking and health: Notions on therapeutic philosophy and philosophical

82

therapy]. In A.-M. Pietilä, T. Hakulinen, E. Hirvonen, P. Koponen, E.-M. Salminen, & K. Sirola (Eds.), *Terveyden edistäminen. Uudistuvat työmenetelmät* [Health promotion. Renewing working methods] (pp. 16-34). Juva: WS Bookwell.

80.   Ryff, C. D., & Singer, B. (1998). Human health: New directions for the next millennium. *Psychological Inquiry, 9,* 69-85.

Educational Viewpoints to Health Promotion among Children and the Youth

How to Use Positive Psychology to Beat Anorexia?

Marika Savukoski, Kaarina Määttä and Satu Uusiautti

Anorexia nervosa is mostly related to different obsessions, an infinite desire to lose weight, and a huge fear of weight gain. Anorectic life seems to just rotate around food and dieting. The secret goal is to destroy one's own appetite completely[1] Life is controlled and over-regulated; repeating the same routines day after day because of the fear of losing control. The anorectic believe that the control shows discipline and self-mastery[2]. In their own eyes, only slenderness and a body without fat appear to validate and offer a decent life[3,4,5]. Anorexia is a business deal grounded in hard thoughts, feelings, and fears, through self punishment[6]. Giddens[7] describes anorexia as a form of addiction in late modern time. He lists the addictions in the anorectic as including coffee, drugs, alcohol, work, fitness, sex, and love. Anorexia demonstrates the negative effect of an individual in society (Giddens, 1996): anorexia enables individuals to try to resolve the question of how to be a good citizen in the performance and efficiency of a society that values them[8].

An estimated 5-10 million girls and women, and nearly a million boys and men, suffer from some form of eating disorder[8]. In Finland, about two percent of women aged between 15 and 20 develop eating disorders and 15 percent have problems with eating[9]. It is one of the most common problems for young women with mental health disorders[10]. In the last decade, according to some research, only about half of the sufferers recover from anorexia[11,12] while in a recent Finnish study, two thirds showed improvement in five years[13]. Some previous studies focusing on beating eating disorders have been conducted[e.g. 14,15,16] but still survival is not guaranteed or the results appear inconsistent [17,18].

The present research gives an extraordinary and unique sight into forms of eating disorders, anorexia, and the enigma of illness and survival from it. The article is based on the interviews of 11 ex-anorectic subjects who each gave their story about their anorectic trip experience and survival. Because of the importance of survival, this research is based on positive psychology as peculiar as it may sound. What could positive psychology offer for the discussion concerning eating disorders, such as anorexia? Anorexia is a serious condition that has to be treated properly—yet the focus of positive psychology is on people's well-being and positive behavioral styles. However, our assumption here is that by paying more attention to the survival stories and the phenomenon of conquering anorexia, we could contribute a positive viewpoint that could help the anorectic and their love ones to struggle and live down anorexia[19]. The article gives hope and strength to believe in healthier tomorrow both to anorectics and their loved ones[e.g. 20].

Therefore, one purpose of the article is to provide the means to survive without losing sight of the difficult fight against anorexia or the painful experiences.

Theoretical Framework

Anorexia and Health

There are several significant typical characteristics of anorexia[21]. The AmericanPsychiatric Association published by definition (DSM-IV) in 1987 the following types:

- A person loses weight to such an extent that their weight drops to at least 15 percent below normal weight.
- There is a personal fear of weight gain and obesity despite the fact that they are already underweight.
- A person considers himself/herself fat although being already abnormally thin.
- Women have amenorrhea and menstruation "opt-out".

Other distinguishing features of anorexia nervosa are hair loss, reduced body temperature, continuous feeling of cold, poor circulation, dry skin, insomnia, nail brittleness, excessive interest in food and calories, low self-esteem, isolation, loneliness, and the inability to concentrate on anything except weight reduction[22,23]. A person diagnosed with anorexia nervosa is classified as having a BMI (Body Mass Index = weight divided by height squared) of less than 17.5[24].

Anorexia is often initiated in adolescence and triggered by new situations in life[19,25]. Impetus for anorexia can come from the simple fear of adolescence. Young people would like to remain young and youthful; avoiding adulthood which brings the inevitable necessity of maturity with menstruation and responsibilities[26,27]. Young people live in the middle of turbulence and seek identity and a place in the world and they have to face their own sexuality and vulnerability[28]. As this kind of crisis develop and make the young feel helpless, they may response to the challenges of society by beginning to destroy themselves through anorexia.

Anorexia is the most extreme response. Becoming anorectic is a form of direction where one turns away from oneself and pursues model citizenship or even something bigger. Anorexia is not comparable with catching a flu and anorectic behavior often starts with sincere aims and commitment to make things right. Their main purpose is to keep transforming into a better person which is thought of being reachable by developing anorexia[e.g.29]. The change does not always imply a deliberate action but it includes anorectic experiences that provide a better situation than the one in the past[6,30]. Maffesoli[31] sees the cure in the adoption of self-turning and self-rescue. Developing anorexia is a sort of call to draw attention to one self and an anorectic person carefully and constantly analyzes the question whether he/she lives sufficiently healthy life, whether his/her weight stays within the limits for an ideal body mass index, and whether he/she is successful in life. Becoming anorectic is a self-absorbed way of living and which – seen through other people's eyes—appears as a very selfish activity[8,30].

Anorexia can be regarded as the "caricatures" of the events that occur when a general recommendation for losing weight is taken too literally and run into the ground. Normal diet becomes scarce and foods, which the anorectic accept, are too healthy[e.g. 32]. The anorectic will remove fat from the diet followed by products containing sugar and this will continue until the only products left are those one containing energy close to zero. Hunger is the maximum enjoyment of the day while eating is such a frightening and distressing experience that persons with anorexia no longer want to be visible to others at the dinner table at the same time[33,34]. Persons with anorexia are unwavering with self-discipline; they are masterful in their eating anxiety when it comes to limiting and not even wanting to taste the "damaging", forbidden food. They are afraid of losing control of themselves if they eat – and therefore, they decide not to eat[2,3]. Eating whatever, however, and at any time is impossible for the anorectic because it violates their "rules"[30]. Still, cooking for others is wonderful because the anorectic enjoy watching others eat. The anorectic collect recipes and walk around the shops to admire the forbidden fruit — the shelves full of delicacies which they do not have the right to consume[33]. In addition, there are plenty of studies that have analyzed the connection between anorexia and suicides and mortality[35,36,37].

Positive Psychology Provides a Positive Attitude toward Life

Interest in themes such as well-being, happiness, quality of life, and positive feelings is germane to positive psychology, a field that has offered studies into the positive characteristics, feelings and strengths of individuals and has also sought to identify phenomena that promote and enhance such positive attributes[38,39]. Gable and Haidt[40] briefly define positive psychology in the following terms: "Positive psychology is the study of the conditions and processes that contribute to the flourishing or optimal functioning of people, groups, and institutions"[40].

The research on the life-span has also contributed to the systematic research on accomplishments and success[39]. The research on happiness has taken root increasingly: in order to know why some people are happier—regardless of the setbacks—than others, we have to understand what the cognitive and motivational processes are that maintain and even increase the happiness and positive attitude[41]. If surviving from anorexia is dissected from a positive perspective, this view is also of great interest. Positive feelings support problem-solving skills and the ability to act in a proactive way. The full importance and potential of this may seem surprising as the emotion of happiness is so simple and common in nature[42]. Positive psychology is also interested in the life spans of positively behaving people and what factors play a key role during the life spans of strong and optimistic people, and how could these factors be recognized? These questions are essential when researching the experiences of beating anorexia.

Well-being is comprehensive social, physical, and emotional experience. It can also be dissected from the point of view of individual strengths that are at the core of positive psychology[39,43] and the focus on human strengths brings positive aspect into well-being and life in general. Seligman and Peterson[44] have analyzed human strengths and how individuals have the possibility to achieve positivity in various life situations. Open mind, critical thinking, and courage, caring for other people, justice, self-regulation, optimism, and hope, among other things, are strengths with which people can achieve well-being[38,45] and should be exploited when struggling with anorexia as well. Therefore, supporting human strengths can enhance, for its part, coping with difficult life situations and events, such as anorexia.

Research Method, Data and Analysis

In this article, our purpose is to dissect the survival stories of those persons who have beaten anorexia: the first and foremost aim is to bring out the factors which made it possible to break free from the anorectic trip. For this reason, one focus of this article is to describe the actual process and models leading to survival. The following question will be answered: What kind of experiences does the process of recovering from anorexia consist of?

The results are considered from the positive point of view. Based on the results, the thought of employing positive psychology in recovering from anorexia will be discussed at the end of the article.

The aim of this research is to understand the reality of anorectic life and related experiences through the individuals' perspective. Those who did get ill are the real experts in describing how they survived. The goal of narrative research is to give subjects the opportunity to make their voices heard because the information which is formed in this way is more polyphonic and varied[e.g. 46]. In this research, participants were Finnish ex-anorectic women (N=11) between the age of 23 and 45 years. They had developed anorexia when between 10 and 18 years old. Each participant's survival story describes their own view of their suffering, disappointments, successes, and joys.

The research participants were selected in this research mostly based on their own willingness to participate. The Finnish Anorexia Association (SYLI) helped in finding the research participants as the first author of this article participates in the action of the association: it informed through its channels of the possibility to participate in this research. Six participants were reached this way. The interviews were designed to concentrate on the interviewees' narration.

Narrative is often associated with the constructivist view of information; reference to the nature of knowledge, knowing, and the process of knowledge itself.

In this study, narrative refers mainly to the nature of the research material and the research data analysis but, equally, it is also research with a constructivist view of knowledge because the examinees themselves have built their knowledge and reality through social interaction[47,48,49]. Silverman[50] points out that research subjects and research tasks for each study are the keys to selecting the most appropriate data collection method. The method in question in this research resembles an application of self-assessment that has been utilized and its reliability has been evaluated in previous researches on anorexia widely[e.g. 51,52]. In this study, the method selected was oral data collection in which the narratives are collected by interviews. In addition, data also consisted of written narratives. The purpose of this study is to describe the participants' survival from anorexia through narratives which have emerged from their personal experiences.

Narrative is also reflected in the method of data analysis which, in this study, was carried out by narrative analysis. In addition, the analysis was also used for categorical content analysis[see 47,53]. Certainly the generalizability, validity, and reliability of the results can be criticized. How truthful are these narratives? They are stories that people who have developed anorexia and beaten it have wanted to bring out afterwards. They represent the truth that the participants have told about their own life. The narratives, thus, include the participants' interpretation of their experiences and they have either consciously or unconsciously withheld some of the experiences, while some other experiences are forgotten and some others are highlighted. Human memory is selective—nor were the participants even able to put everything into words[54]. However, those narratives that they have told voluntarily involve valuable information as such and form a reality of their own[55,56].

Results

Recovering from anorexia can be viewed as a development conversion during which persons with anorexia begin to observe the world around them in new ways making anorexia gradually disappear. The process is slow because they will have to re-learn the so-called normal life. Healing should involve long-term projects of experimental and internal discovery during which it is acceptable to fail and grope towards success[20]. It is important to remember that the way to a flat stomach is through a swollen belly and that the healing process, caused by anxiety and the presence of evil, comes after the freedom that allows the head to shatter the twisted thoughts and myths[57].

> "Survival, it's like learning to read, because you have to be extremely careful in all the phases and steps not to fall apart, and then you had to slowly and carefully think over all the things: to cram, repeat, and practice. You had to feed information into yourself and those new schemes of things…"

When talking about their survival, the participants emphasized their spiritual survival stories and their analyzing methods—the processes through which each became anorectic or mindful of their initial experiences and feelings. These social supports aimed at finding the ways of coping with the emotional state and providing the ultimate aim of reducing the internal stress caused by emotional discomfort[58].

> "I had to learn that if someone feels bad it is not necessarily my fault at all. Or if someone has done wrong, I don't have to go and fix it immediately. I learned that you have a right to feel things and you don't have to hide them but, you know, to accept them."

In practice, a known key to the survival is trying to work on negative emotions such as hatred, anger, and bitterness as well as learning about the lives of others who have had such feelings. Equally, it is a question of forgetting, forgiving, and finding meaning in their painful experiences[59,60]. The extent of an individual's internal stress-regulatory refers mainly to the abilities of elimination, problem solving, emotional processing, and partly also the control of the above mentioned. When beating anorexia, persons with anorexia are not able to change their life but they have to change themselves. Giddens[61] calls this approach to anorectic survival the idea of an identity project during which the persons with anorexia are reflective and re-evaluate them in order to continue efforts for survival. Yet, it is important to allow time for setbacks and occasional returns to anorectic life as the healing is not always—if ever—straightforward.

> "For me, survival is more like becoming harmonious, like sewing the wounds and fixing the scarves engraved in your mind; those scarves that had been opened by all the comments, twitting, and insults. I learned to think from a whole new perspective and tried to see myself in a whole new light, too."

The key to struggling against anorexia seems to be emphasizing the practical means to influence the situation or the ways to get help for oneself. Lazarus and Folkman[59] tested these problem-based methods along with Endler and Parker[60] for task-oriented survival. These methods of testing included enrollment in public health care, school health care, or peer groups. Sports, hobbies, and sometimes the use of pharmaceuticals proved to be successful in solving problems[62, see also 32,63,64].

> "It relieved me in a big way. I could talk the monster out of my head; and that psychologist who luckily happened to be a great person was the most helpful. Namely, I have heard afterwards that quite many, equal to me, have had really bad experiences on the psychologists and their ways of action..."

"There [at yoga] I became acquainted with my own body and its needs. And that put my mind at rest too... Since, I have done some jogging and swimming as well but that yoga has become a permanent hobby for me."

Beating anorexia appears to be driven by both the spiritual survival of the process, whose main objective is to reach and overcome the emotions caused by the anorectic experiences and by learning to live with these feelings. It also involves practical problem solving means, such as seeking outside assistance[62]. However, it also affects survival attitudes in the physical environment and the challenges of everyday living including how a person may combine work, study, and family life. It is important to note that the survival in each case may be very different for different individuals. A person may feel that a particular way of survival is good and meaningful while the method employed could be seen by outsiders as redundant and inefficient[65]. Therefore, the evaluation of the effectiveness of survival is not in priority since an individual's own experience of survival is more important: whether the decisive step is in an active role of changing the situation or a passive one such as treatment[59,66].

In this research, the aim was to find out what coping factors helped the persons with anorexia to find what is missing in their lives or how they survived as winners against the tough opponent of anorexia. There is more than one reason for developing anorexia and the same can be said about survival. Coping, for an individual, is the sum of several factors including the available resources, their strengths, previous life history, social status, and personality. This research, therefore, is just the beginning and adds another voice to those authors who have broken through the strong and protective wall which surrounds anorexia.

In this research the survivors had clear similarities which were repeated in almost every survival story. One such similarity was toughness—a characteristic perceived as striving in spite of adversity until the goal is reached. Persistence is also linked to a commitment and confidence in the target being achievable[45]. According to Eisenberg and Wang[67], the persistence of people is also able to help regulate their own behavior ranges which increases the persistent human adaptability, holistic well-being, and functioning. The survivors in this research proved to be persistent: at first they changed their lives very systematically, without giving up, toward a complete state of anorexia and then, later, they used that same tenacity to return back to a somewhat normal life. The disease, therefore, already demonstrated that the participants were tenacious when faced with a goal and but even more perseverant by surviving the many uphill battles faced after a long healing process.

"...but then I was thinking it over for a long time; that now the case is that I can't do this darn thinking any longer, that it is now or never: Either I decide that I will die or then I carry on living and actually do something. So then, I decided that I still want to live and get better really..."

Starting over was clearly one similar feature among the participants. It was reflected, above all, in the wider opportunities which invaded and changed their old, anorectic thoughts and eating habits by setting up small safety lines for a new life. Survival was also reflected in the changing of relationships, changes in the place of residence, relaxation of self-discipline, and also learning how to use relaxation and laziness. Putting things aside was a necessary strategy; a case of throwing overboard the whole anorectic life and taking up almost everything from scratch.

> "...I really started to think about what I actually think of this and that, whether I want to go there, what kinds of people I like, and, you know, about all ordinary things. I think that all started from zero; I am ashamed to tell that I had to learn again how to brush my teeth, because at that time, I was so depressed that I couldn't do things like that."

On the other hand, the survivors needed time to manage both the journey and the trade-offs as carefully as possible. They needed the space and time to grow as well as the opportunity to develop and build their own identity in the imperfect world. Wenger[68] mentioned the idea of the individual's inner dialogue about becoming and avoiding something. The persons with anorexia would construct their identities during coping or through social relations and by using various entities such as peer support groups[49,68]. Recovering from anorexia nervosa represents, therefore, a kind of growth. It requires maturation of ideas and comprehensive self-acceptance, mostly in adult life, as they have often developed anorexia already during a developmental crisis in their adolescence. Growth is also linked to improved self-esteem which is shown, above all, in self-respect and the success of social relationships[69].

> "In my opinion, the conversation itself with those who had experienced the same is really a good thing. If you explained these things to someone who hasn't experienced it, it would be almost the same as talking to walls... When you have a talk with someone with the same experiences, it feels wonderful when you don't need to explain what you mean if you said aloud that 'darn how distressed I am'."

Beating anorexia is comparable with the idea of surviving and one of the desired outcomes is to achieve good life-management skills. The road to good life management consists of efforts to focus on causes, deploy information and advice, find a positive attitude to life, and make the use of already existing or newly-born internal strengths consciously. By using the strength of the classification developed by Fernández-Ballesteros[70], the key survival factors among the participants in this research were optimism, internal motivation, personality development, social network and support, social opportunities, and partly confidence in aptitude, wisdom and happiness [see also 36].

Optimism was reflected in all of these examined factors as well as the courage to turn away from the familiar and safe in order to seize new life challenges[71]. Internal motivation resembled the participants' personal desire to survive and achieve sustainable improvements in life. Internal motivation describes, therefore, an individual's need to learn and develop but it also contains one's personality structure and motivation to develop[72,73]. The subjects had self-realization which opened the way to turn from anorectic thoughts and provided the opportunity to enjoy a life of sport, art, animals, or music. Social support was considered an opportunity to talk about the difficulties and contradictions with someone else but also a channel to get new information about the problem. Furthermore, social support enabled the anorectic to request assistance and experience the feeling of security[13,74]. Social contacts opened up opportunities to visualize a normal life and reflect on distorted perceptions.

"She [a friend] has been able to be by my side the whole time and when I was in a bad shape, she would be in contact with me all the time and ask how I am doing. She also understands me in that sense well, because she has had the same kinds of experiences; however, just a little bit different situation than mine is. You know, we can understand each other more easily and we don't face a situation where one would consider the other stupid after acting in some insane way ever. Both understand that this action might not be conscious but there is a reason for it."

Happiness was revealed and, above all, when acquired through the love of either a spouse or a child created the power to remain and survive. True love, which was based on happiness, gave the participants an opportunity to grow as a person and meet their goals[75]. Self-examination awoke confidence through both the ability and the crucial experience of surviving an attainable goal. Maddux[76] notes that personal faith in achieving the goal is one of the most important factors that lead to success. All of these strengths are basic wisdom and reflect the internal resources examined and detected in the study for the adjustment of life's tensions and seeing the puzzle piece by piece[77].

"..I still don't know why I didn't die from these medications. Neither could anyone else explain it to me. I have been thinking myself that it wasn't my time to go yet and this information gave me a lot of strength... Therefore, in the middle of feeling so powerful, there in the hospital, I decided that I will end anorexia, not myself..."

Conclusions and Discussion

People who have beaten anorexia find it often difficult to name the exact factors that have brought them toward survival[e.g. 14,15,16,17,18]. Anorectic time consists of painful memories; which is good because, otherwise, the continuation of life would be really difficult. However, it also makes the survival difficult as some experiences can be completely ignored and concealed. The coping factors which were found in this research may somehow generate understanding about those types through which survival is possible and these results are mostly exemplary approaches to anorexia. Furthermore, based on the results, we encourage people who help the persons with anorexia to take into account the individual's life as a whole rather than offering them a pre-packed, particular or existing model of treatment. Thus, recovering from anorexia cannot be described through any particular model or strategy because the underlying models of individuals facing the coping task meet many twists, turns, or pauses. After all, survival consists of good luck and happiness as well as being aware of different coping models through which the motivation to survive will be aroused.

Recovering anorexia seems to be both art and science: Science in the sense that the persons with anorexia have invented ways to deal with the state of malnutrition and art in the sense that any treatment depends of the situation, personality, and experience and is unique. Large, ad hoc approaches, due to differences in treatments, are not for everyone[33] and predicting the result can be difficult because patients do not want treatment. Particularly difficult and long-lasting therapy will often go hand in hand with other problems such as obsessive and compulsive disorder, anxiety disorder, personality disorder, major depressive disorder, massive fatigue, confusion, thoughts of suicide, family problems, alcohol, drugs, and medicine abuse[12,78,79]. Recovering from anorexia nervosa is not a miracle but mostly a long, unpleasant, and complicated journey toward an internal and external transformation. Treatments are extremely important forms of support and security to persons with anorexia who are directed in a new journey [see also 80].

In this article, we wanted to pay special attention to the positive approach of beating anorexia. It was possible through the participants' survival stories as the aim was to bring out positive elements that help struggling with anorexia and that could be of use both for persons with anorexia and their loved ones. Focusing on personal strengths and finding the positive attitude toward the change away from the anorectic life and—the most importantly—toward oneself, appeared difficult but crucial means to survival. In counseling and psychotherapy and clinical psychology, applied positive psychology builds on the traditions of humanistic psychology and promotes a dimensional understanding of mental health and mental illness by, for example, contributing happiness-increase interventions, such as using signature strengths, person-centered approach and positive therapy, and life coaching[81]. At the subjective level, positive psychology concentrates on subjective experiences, well-being, satisfaction, flow, joy, pleasure, and happiness, as well as on optimistic and hopeful attitude and confidence in the future. At the group level, the interest is on the civil skills and institutions that make the individuals turn into better citizens—responsible, flexible, and ethical people[82]. In future, it would be interesting to conduct interventions that are based on positive psychology and at the institutional level to analyze how anorexia could be prevented or how its treatment could be enhanced by functional and health-promoting institutions.

References

1. Miller, C. A., & Golden N. H. (2010). An introduction to eating disorders: Clinical presentation, epidemiology, and prognosis. *Nutrition in Clinical Practice, 25*(2), 110-115.
2. Bissada, H., Tasca, G. A., Marber, A. M., & Bradwejn, J. (2008). Olanzapine in the treatment of low body weight and obsessive thinking in women with anorexia nervosa: A randomized, double-blind, placebo-contolled trial. *The American Journal of Psychiatry, 165*(10), 1281-1288.
3. Bordo, S. (1993). *Unbearable weight. Feminism, western culture and body.* Berkeley, CA: University of California Press.
4. Mussell, P. M., Mitchell, J. E., & Binford, R. B. (2001). Anorexia Nervosa. In J. E. Mitchell (Ed.), *Outpatient treatment of eating disorder: A guide for therapist, dieticians and physicians* (pp. 5-25). Minnesota: University of Minnesota Press.
5. Schooler, D. (2008). Real women have curves: a longitudinal investigation of TV and the body image development of Latina adolescents. *Journal of Adolescent Research, 23*(2), 132-153.
6. Puuronen, A. (2004a). *Rasvan tyttäret. Etnografinen tutkimus anorektisen kokemustiedon kulttuurisesta jäsentymisestä* [Daughters of fat. Ethnographic research of anorectic knowledge gained from experience of cultural organization]. Helsinki: Hakapaino.
7. Giddens, A. (1996). Life in post-traditional society. In U. Beck, A. Giddens, & S. Lash (Eds.), *Modern track. Reflexive modernization* (pp. 83-152). Cambridge: Polity Press.
8. Michel, D. M., & Willard, S. G. (2003). *When dieting becomes dangerous. A guide to understanding and treating anorexia and bulimia.* Yale: Yale University Press.
9. Ruuska, J. (2006). *The impact of eating disorders on the adolescent process.* Tampere: Tampere University Press.
10. Yager, J., Devlin, M. J., Halmi, K. A., & Zerbe K. J. (2005). Eating disorders. *Focus, 3*(4), 503-510.
11. Zandian, M., Ioakimidis, I., Bergh, C., & Södersten, P. (2007). Cause and treatment of Anorexia Nervosa. *Physiology & Behavior, 92*(1-2), 283-290.
12. Seller, C. A., & Ravalia, A. (2003). Anaesthetic implications of anorexia nervosa. *Anesthetic, 58*(5), 437-443.
13. Keski-Rahkonen, A., Hoek, H. W., Susser, E. S., & Rissanen, A. (2007). Epidemiology and course of anorexia nervosa in the community. *American Journal of Psychiatry, 164*(8), 1259-1265.
14. Lindblad, F., Lindberg, L., & Hjern, A. (2006). Improved survival in adolescent patients with anorexia nervosa: a comparison of two Swedish national cohorts of female inpatients. *The American Journal of Psychiatry, 163*(8), 1433-1435.
15. Wagner, A., Aizenstein, H., Venkatraman, V. K., & Kaye, W. H. (2007). Altered reward processing in women recovered from anorexia nervosa. *The American Journal of Psychiatry, 164*(12), 1842-1849.
16. Weaver, K., Wuest, J., & Ciliska, D. (2005). Understanding women's journey of recovering from anorexia nervosa. *Qualitative Health Research, 15*(2), 188-206.

17.   Bulik, C. M. (2002). One half of patients with anorexia nervosa fully recovered after 21 years but the other half had a chronic or lethal course. *Evidence Based Mental Health, 5*(2), 59.

18.   Sullivan, P. F. (2003). Discrepant results regarding long-term survival of patients with anorexia nervosa? *Mayo Clinic Proceedings, 78*(3), 273-274.

19.   Swanson, S. A., Crow, S. J., Le Grange, D., Swendsen, J., & Merikangas, K. R. (2011). Prevalence and correlates of eating disorders in adolescents: results from the national comorbidity survey replication adolescent supplement. *Archive of General Psychiatry, 68*(7), 714-723.

20.   Sim, L. A., McAlpine, D. E., Grothe, K. B., & Clark, M. M. (2010). Identification and treatment of eating disorders in the primary care setting. *Mayo Clinic Proceedings, 85*(8), 746-751.

21.   Attia, E., & Walsh, B. T. (2007). Anorexia Nervosa. *The American Journal of Psychiatry, 164*(12), 1805-1810.

22.   Bryant-Waugh, R. (2006). Recent developments in Anorexia Nervosa. *Child and Adolescent Mental Health, 11*(2), 76-81.

23.   Duker, M., & Slade, R. (2003). *Anorexia Nervosa and Bulimia. How to help.* Buckingham: Open University Press.

24.   Abraham, S., & Llewellyn-Jones, D. (2001). *Eating disorders. The facts.* Oxford: Oxford University Press.

25.   Engblom, P. (1998). *Naisen itsekokemus, identiteetti ja psykodynaaminen psykoterapia syömishäiriöissä* [Woman's experience of self, identity and psychodynamic psychotherapy in eating disorders]. Helsinki: Hakapaino.

26.   Charpentier, P. (1998). Anoreksia ja bulimia [Anorexia and Bulimia]. In P. Charpentier (Ed.), *Nuorten syömishäiriöt ja lihavuus* [Young people's eating disorders and obesity] (pp. 7-24). Jyväskylä: Kirjapaino Oma.

27.   Lawson, E. A., Miller, K. K., Mathur, V. A., Misra, M., Meenaghan, E., Herzog, D. B., & Klibanski, A. (2007). Hormonal and nutritional effects on cardiovascular risk markers in young women. *The Journal of Clinical Endocrinology & Metabolism, 92*(8), 3089-3094.

28.   Jaffe, K., & Worobey, J. (2006). Mothers' attitudes toward fat, weight and dieting in themselves and their children. *Body Image, 3*(2), 113-120.

29.   Hurley, R. A., & Taber, K. H. (2008). Imaging of eating disorders: multiple techniques to demonstrate the dynamic brain. *The Journal of Neuropsychiatry and Clinical Neurosciences, 20*(3), iv-260.

30.   Puuronen, A (2004b). Anoreksia uskontotieteen tutkimuskentällä [Anorexia in the field of religion science]. In O. Fingerroos, M. Opas, & T. Taira (Eds.), *Uskonnon paikka. Kirjoituksia uskontojen ja uskontoteorioiden rajoista* [Place of religion. Writings of the limits of religions and religious theories]. Helsinki: Hakapaino.

31.   Maffesoli, M. (1995). *Maailman mieli: yhteisöllisen tyylin muodoista* [The world's mind:collaborative style formats]. Helsinki: Gaudeamus.

32.   Muller, W. (2009). Towards research-based approaches for solving body composition problems in sports: Ski jumping as a heuristic example. *British Journal of Sports Medicine, 43*(13), 1013-1019.

33.   Lucas, A. R. (2004). *Demystifying anorexia nervosa: an optimistic guide to understanding and healing.* Oxford: Oxford University Press.

34.   Thurfjell, B. (2005). *Adolescent eating disorders in a socio-cultural context.* Uppsala: Uppsala University.

35.   Bulik, C. M., Thornton, L., Poyastro Pinheiro, A., Kaye, W. H. (2008). Suicide attempts in Anorexia Nervosa. *Psychosomatic Medicine, 70*(3), 378-383.

36.   Kaye, W. (2009). Eating disorders: hope despite mortal risk. *The American Journal of Psychiatry, 166*(12), 1309-1311.

37.   Papadopoulos, F. C., Ekbom, L., Brandt, L., & Ekselius, L. (2009). Excess mortality, causes of death and prognostic factors in anorexia nervosa. *The British Journal of Psychiatry, 194*(1), 10-17.

38.   Seligman, M. E. P., Steen, T. A., Park, N., & Peterson, C. (2005). Positive psychology progress. Empirical validation of interventions. *American Psychologist, 60*, 410-421.

39.   Aspinwall, L. G., & Staudinger, U. M. (Eds.) (2003). *A psychology of human strengths: Fundamental questions and future directions for a positive psychology.* San Francisco, CA: Berrett-Koehler.

40.   Gable, S., & Haidt, J. (2005). What (and why) is positive psychology? *Review of General Psychology, 9*, 103-110.

41.   Lyubomirsky, S. (2001). Why are some people happier than others? The role of cognitive and motivational processes in well-being. *American Psychologist, 56*, 239-249.

42.   Isen, A. M. (2006). Myönteinen tunne ihmisen vahvuuden lähteenä [Positive feeling as a source of human strength]. In L. G. Aspinwall & U. M. Staudinger (Eds.), *Ihmisen vahvuuksien psykologia* [A psychology of human strengths] (pp. 186-201). Helsinki: Edita.

43.   Carruthers, C., & Hood, C. D. (2005). The power of positive psychology. *Parks & Recreation, Oct 2005*, 30-37.

44.   Seligman, M. E. P., & Peterson, C. (2003). Positive clinical psychology. In L. Aspinwall & U. Staudinger (Eds.), *A Psychology of human strengths. Fundamental questions and future directions for a positive psychology* (pp. 305-317). Washington, DC: American Psychological Association.

45.   Carver, C. S., & Scheier, M. F. (2003). Three human strengths. In L. G. Aspinwall & U. M. Staudinger (Eds.), *A psychology of human strengths: Fundamental questions and future directions for a positive psychology* (pp. 87-102). San Francisco, CA: Berrett-Koehler.

46.   Holloway, I. (2011). Being a qualitative researcher. *Qualitative Health Research, 21*(7), 968-975.

47.   Lieblich, A., Tuval-Machiach, R., & Zilber, T. (1998). *Narrative research: Reading, analysis and interpretation.* Thousand Oaks, CA: Sage.

48.   Garro, C., & Mattingly, L. C. (2000). *Narrative and the cultural construction of illness and healing.* Berkeley, CA: University of California Press.

49.   Mahoney, M. J. (2002). Constructivism and positive psychology. In C. R. Snyder & S. J. Lopez (Eds.), *Handbook of positive psychology* (pp. 745-750). Oxford: University Press.

50.   Silverman, D. (2005). *Doing qualitative research.* London: Sage.

51.   Rathner, G., & Rumpold, G. (2006). Convergent validity of the eating disorder inventory and the anorexia nervosa inventory for self-rating in an Austrian nonclinical population. *International Journal of Eating Disorders, 16*(4), 381-193.

52.   Schoemaker, C., van Strien, T., & van der Staak, C. (1994). Validation of the eating disorders inventory in a nonclinical population using transformed and untransformed responses. *International Journal of Eating Disorders, 15*(4), 387-393.

53.   Polkinghorne, D. (1995). Narrative configuration in qualitative analysis. In J. A. Hatch & R. Wisniewski (Eds.), *Life history and narrative* (pp. 5-24). London: Falmer.

54.   Buchbinder, E. (2011). Beyond checking. Experiences of the validation interview. *Qualitative Social Work, 10*(1), 106-122.

55.   Whittemore, R., Chase, S., & Mandle, C. L. (2001). Validity in qualitative research. *Qualitative Health Research, 11*(4), 522-537.

56.   Wuest, J. (2011). Are we there yet? Positioning qualitative research differently. *Qualitative Health Research, 21*(7), 875-883.

98

57.   Ster, G. V. D. (2006). *Lupa syödä. Opas syömishäiriöiden hoitoon* [License to eat. Guide to eating disorders treatment]. Helsinki: Edita Prima.
58.   Hogh, A., & Dofradottir, A. (2001). Coping with bullying in the workplace. *European Journal of Work and Organizational Psychology, 10*(4), 485-495.
59.   Lazarus, R. S., & Folkman, S. (1984). *Stress, appraisal and coping.* New York, NY: Springer.
60.   Endler, N. S., & Parker, J. D. A. (1994). Assessment of multidimensional coping: task, emotion and avoidance strategies. *Psychological Assessment, 6*(1), 50-60.
61.   Giddens, A. (1991). *Modernity and self-identity. Self and society in the late modern age.* Cambridge: Polity Press.
62.   Latack, J. C., & Havlovic, S. J. (1992). A conceptual evaluation framework for coping measures. *Journal of Organizational Behavior, 13*(5), 479-508.
63.   Jackson, C. W., Cates, M., & Lorenz, R. (2010). Pharmacotherapy of eating disorders. *Nutrition in Clinical Practice, 25*(2), 143-159.
64.   Rossi, G., Balottin, U., Rossi, M., & Lanzi, G. (2007). Pharmacological treatment of anorexia nervosa: a retrospective study in preadolescents and adolescents. *Clinical Pediatrics, 46*(9), 806-811.
65.   Vitaliano, P., Maieiro, R., Russo, I., Katon, W., & Hall, G. (1990). Coping profiles associated with psychiatric, physical health, work, and family problems. *Health Psychology, 9*(3), 348-376.
66.   Rajala, R. (2001). *Stressinhallinta opettajien kertomuksissa: onnistunut ja epäonnistunut stressinhallinta kouluyhteisössä* [Stress management teacher reports: successful and unsuccessful stress management in the school community]. Rovaniemi: University of Lapland.
67.   Eisenberg, N., & Wang, V. O. (2003). Toward a positive psychology: Social developmental and cultural contributions. In L. G. Aspinwall & U. M. Staudinger (Eds.), *A psychology of human strengths: Fundamental questions and future directions for a positive psychology* (pp. 117-129). San Francisco, CA: Berrett-Koehler.
68.   Wenger, E. (2002). Communities of practice and social learning systems. In F. Reeve, M. Carrewright, & R. Edwards (Eds.), *Supporting lifelong learning 2: organizing learning* (pp. 160-179). London & New York: RoutledgeFalmer.
69.   Mäkikangas, A. (2007). *Personality, well-being and job resources. From negative paradigm towards positive psychology.* Jyväskylä: Jyväskylä University Printing House.
70.   Fernández-Ballesteros, R. (2003). Light and dark in the psychology of human strengths: The example of psychogerontology. In L. G. Aspinwall & U. M. Staudinger (Eds.), *A psychology of human strengths: Fundamental questions and future directions for a positive psychology* (pp. 131-147). San Francisco, CA: Berrett-Koehler.
71.   Folkman, S., Lazarus, R. S., Dunkel-Schetter, C., DeLongis, A., & Gruen, R. J. (1986). Dynamics of a stressful encounter outcomes. *Journal of Personality and Social Psychology, 50*(5), 992-1003.
72.   Nurmi, J.-E., & Salmela-Aro, K. (2006). What works make you happy: The role of personal goals in life-span development. In M. Csikszentmihalyi & I. S. Csikszentmihalyi (Eds.), *Life worth living: Contributions of positive psychology* (pp. 182-199). Oxford: Oxford University Press.
73.   Ryan, R. M., & Deci, E. L. (2000). Self-determination theory and the facilitation of intrinsic motivation, social development and well-being. *American Psychologist, 55*(1), 68-78.
74.   Scheff, T. (1990). *Microsociology. Discourse, emotion, and social structure.* London: The University of Chicago Press.

75.   Hendricks, S., & Hendricks, C. (2002). Love. In C. R. Snyder & S. J. Lopez (Eds.), *Handbook of positive psychology* (pp. 472-484). Oxford: Oxford University Press.

76.   Maddux, J. E. (2002). Self-Efficacy. The power of believing you can. In C. R. Snyder & S. J. Lopez (Eds.), *Handbook of positive psychology* (pp. 277-287). Oxford: Oxford University Press.

77.   Baltes, P. B., & Freund, A. M. (2003). Human strengths as the orchestrations of wisdom and selective optimization with compensation. In L. G. Aspinwall & U. M. Staudinger (Eds.), *A psychology of human strengths: Fundamental questions and future directions for a positive psychology* (pp. 23-35). San Francisco, CA: Berrett-Koehler.

78.   Lock, J., et al. (2010). Randomized clinical trial comparing family-based treatment with adolescent-focused individual therapy for adolescents with anorexia nervosa. *Archives of General Psychiatry, 67*(10), 1025-1032.

79.   McIntosh, V. V. W. (2005). Three psychoterapies for anorexia nervosa: a randomized, controlled trial. *The American Journal of Psychiatry, 162*(4), 741-747.

80.   Savukoski, M., Määttä, K., & Uusiautti, S. (2011). The other side of well-being-what makes a young woman become an anorectic? *International Journal of Psychological Studies, 3*(2), 76-86.

81.   Linley, P. A., Joseph, S., Maltby, J., Harrington, S., & Wood, A. M. (2009). Positive psychology applications. In S. J. Lopez & C. R. Snyder (Eds.), *Oxford handbook of positive psychology* (pp. 35-47). Oxford: Oxford University Press,.

82.   Seligman, M. E. P. (2002). Positive psychology, positive prevention, and positive therapy. In C. R. Snyder & S. J. Lopez (Eds.), *Handbook of positive psychology* (pp. 3-9). Oxford: Oxford University Press.

How to Overcome Bullying at School?

Sanna Hoisko, Satu Uusiautti and Kaarina Määttä

Bullying is an unfortunate part of humanity: it occurs in the human relationships and therefore, also at school. Bullying is a subtype of aggressive behavior, in which an individual or a group of individuals repeatedly attacks, humiliates, and/or excludes a relatively powerless person [1]. Bullying as a phenomenon is widely studied in a variety of disciplines during the past few decades[see 1,2,3,4]. More and more expressions of violence and malaise take place in schools and youth camps[see also 5,6] —even in the form of ultimate violence, massacre, as happened for example in Norway (July 2011) and Finland (November 2007) traditionally considered as "lands of milk and honey". In Finland, bullying at school has drawn increasing attention since the massacres as bullying was found as one of the background factors in these events. There are differences in the prevalence of bullying within countries[3]; yet, between 8–54% of school-age children become victims of bullying according to international studies[7,8].

There are numerous interventions and methods to prevent and stop bullying at school[e.g. 4] but still the number of victims is countless. In this study, the focus is on the victims' perception on their coping methods. Particularly, researchers will study adult ex- victims' experiences. Bullying may destroy its victim's life but there are also success stories about people who have survived and even succeeded in their life after being bullied at school.

Therefore, the perspective researchers take on bullying is fundamentally positive and will discuss the phenomenon of bullying at school grounding on the ideas from positive psychology[9,10]. Why do some people survive better than others and how do they cope with bullying? The only way of revealing such positive coping strategies is, according to the principles of positive psychology[11,12], to study people who have survived and are willing to discuss their experiences.

Perspectives on Bullying

Many researchers have defined the concept of bullying. Norwegian Dan Olweus[13], who is considered as a pioneer of bullying research[see 3], emphasized the repetitive nature of bullying. According to a Finnish researcher Christina Salmivalli[1], the concept of bullying is used for referring to peer-to-peer bullying among school-aged children and youth, when not otherwise mentioned. The key features of bullying include the intent to harm, the repeated aspect of the harmful acts, and the power imbalance between bully and victims[4].

Furthermore, victims of bullying can be defined in a variety of ways. Victims of bullying can be classified into subgroups for example according to whether or not they bully others as well: pure victims are children who are solely victims of bullies, and bully/victims are children who are simultaneously victims of bullies and bully[2]. In addition to the bully and victim, bullying process involves students who take on other roles (called participant roles): assistants of the bully, reinforcers of the bully, defenders of the victim, and outsiders[see 3,14]. Indeed, Swedish Researcher Anatol Pikas considered bullying as group violence because it is an attack against an individual[15]. However, it is crucial to understand that bullying is a subjective experience. Everyone experiences it in a personal way: while someone can interpret bullying as a playful teasing, some other could consider the same kind of behavior quite defamatory bullying[16,17,18].

One way of analyzing the forms of bullying is to divide it into direct and indirect bullying. For example, hitting, kicking, pushing, tingling, and calling somebody names are direct bullying. Indirect bullying takes the form of ridiculing, social rejection, or spreading rumors of someone. The latter is usually difficult to detect but even when it is obvious it might be difficult to recognize[14]. In addition physical, verbal, and social types of bullying can be distinguished[19]. Various forms of bullying have been reported already at pre- school level [see e.g. 20,21]. Along with advances in information technology, a new form of bullying has occurred: cyber bullying. Bullying by the internet and mobile phones may have countlessly bystanders because emails, pictures, and videos can easily be shared with millions of people. Through the internet, a bully can reach his or her victim at home and thus, bullying is not limited only at school or on school commutes but can take place 24/7 [22, see also 23]. The reasons for starting bullying often hark back to time before going to school[e.g. 24]. Nowadays, instead of personal matters, more attention is paid to peer-group qualities[25]. It has been noticed that bullying is likely to occur in groups that lack genuine sense of togetherness and cohesion as this kind of atmosphere makes the bully's aggressive and domineering behavior possible[26,27].

Select Coping Theories

Crises and hardships in life can cause stress, a state of imbalance in mental, social, and/or physical life that one has to cope with[28]. Bullying at school represents such a situation. When people talk about coping or survival, they usually refer to surviving from something bad. In addition, survival is a personal experience of coping[29].

According to Furman[30], people tend to perceive their past and suffering merely as a strength than a negative factor. Understanding enhances coping. If the victim understands and does not blame him or herself, he or she has the possibility to survive. A positive attitude certainly boosts the healing process[11]. According to Heiskanen[31], the process of coping can be surprisingly long and that usually needs some kind of impetus to begin.

In this research, theory presented by Ayalon[32] about coping is in the center. Every human being has his or her own kind or way of coping that includes typical habits and aptitudes in facing the challenges of life. Ayalon's theory consists of six dimensions that are beliefs and values, emotions, social interaction, imagination, cognitions, and the physiological dimension. Everyone possesses all these dimensions and uses them as a unique, personal combination in the coping process.

Cullberg[33] distinguishes several phases in coping with traumatic events: the phase of shock, reaction, processing, and taking the new direction. Coping is regarded as a journey that does not necessarily pass all of the above-mentioned phases: a phase can be totally missed or can occur simultaneously with some other phase. Cullberg's theory can be seen as a means for helping someone in crisis.

Bullying is a long-term phenomenon and continuous but single bullying events are sudden and unexpected that cause feelings similar to the phase of shock. The purpose of this phase is to protect human mind from unbearable information or experience, for example by denial[33, see also 34]. Some crises start by degrees so that one may not experience an actual shock. Bullying can represent such an event and the process of coping could start straight from the second phase; that is the phase of reaction. This phase usually arouses powerful emotions, such as anger and fear, when the dangerous situation is already over. In this phase, people tend to find a meaning for what happened and to discuss the experience. In the phase of processing the trauma, the victim of bullying starts to analyze the situation and, little by little, accepts it[33]. The purpose of this phase is to work with negative feelings which can be enhanced by, for example, reading and writing[34]. The final phase is to find the new direction. The victim begins to heal and see life without the pain caused by bullying. Forgiveness is a part of this phase. It is reasonable to talk about survival when bullying does not occupy one's mind constantly nor does thinking about it cause anxiety and fear. Instead, that phase of life can calmly be perceived as a part of oneself, an experience that one has gone through[33,34].

Method

Bullying is a phenomenon that concerns many people. The purpose of this research is to find out—from the adult survivors' perspective—how victims of bullying have survived and what kinds of coping methods they have used. The main research question is the following: What kinds of coping methods have the victims of bullying used to overcome bullying?

A qualitative research approach was selected to study this serious phenomenon and to acquire survivors' perceptions and experiences[35]. Thus, the purpose was not to draw any statistical conclusions but to understand adult survivors' coping strategies and ways as comprehensively as possible[36].

The data for this research were collected from open Finnish internet forums where people can write about their experiences of bullying anonymously. Internet forums represent interactive social interaction and the messages in the forums are often characterized as written speech as they seemingly can be defined to be somewhere between speech and text. Internet forums are clearly products of the modern culture and numerous issues are discussed 24/7[see 37].Seven chains of messages were selected from three forums. The criterion for selection was based on either the title of the messages or the content of the first message in the chain. The longest chain consisted of 80 messages and the shortest of five messages. Altogether, the data consisted of 190 messages written by 142 pseudonyms.

Because of the pseudonyms, it is impossible to know who the actual people behind the writings are. However, based on the information and hints revealed in messages, it was possible to draw some kind of a picture, for example, about the participants' gender, age, and professions. The age of the writers could be interpreted from their comments on working life, retirement and grandchildren, their own children, and the form of pseudonym (e.g. Pirjo27 could refer to the writer's first name and age). Some of them revealed their age within the message text. Thirty- three were identified as women and eight as men. The rest of the writers did not mention their gender. Table 1 illustrates the age distribution in this study.

Table 1. The participants' ages

Age (years)	Number of pseudonyms (n)
11–20	4
21–30	14
12	2
41–50	5
Age undefinable	107
Total	142

Despite the above-mentioned deficiencies, internet forums provide a chance to express one's opinion in public and get feedback[38]. Therefore, forums enable interaction with other people and can have an important impact in the lives of those people who participate in discussions. Because of anonymity, it is possible to discuss even the most difficult issues with other people. Therefore, people can reveal their most hidden feelings and talk about their dubious coping methods that they might have used. It is possible that this kind of information would not be revealed for example in interviews.

The data were analyzed through qualitative content analysis which can be divided into theory- bound, theory-based, or data-based content analysis. The theory-based analysis is based on some certain theory, model, or idea and research follows this select model, first by describing the theory and then by using the core concepts as the theoretical framework. This research has features of both theory and data-based analyses. On the other hand, the data were analyzed by its content in order to find the most distinctive categories in it. However, the coping methods found in the data resemble Ayalon[32] six-dimensional coping theory. Therefore, coping methods and strategies were eventually categorized (retelling Ayalon's theory) into the following categories:

(1) Cognitive coping methods
(2) Emotional coping methods
(3) Social coping methods
(4) Creative coping methods
(5) Physiological coping methods
(6) Spiritual coping methods

Results

In this data, coping was fundamentally perceived in two ways: either survival equaled the end of bullying or when the trauma caused by bullying was treated. In general, survival was seen as a desirable target and an ideal state. However, it is a process that may not necessarily become ever finished. The status of victim does not disappear and one has to go through all lost things that cause bitterness and hatred before healing can begin. Some people can heal quickly while others' healing processes lasts longer[39]. Several coping methods were found in the messages written in the internet forums. The results are introduced according to the categories introduced in Method chapter.

Cognitive Coping Methods

One natural coping method is to defend oneself. It, however, requires boldness and self- confidence, features that long-term bullying is likely to extirpate from the victim sooner or later. Eventually, the victim of bullying may not know how or does not have the courage to defend any longer. When the victim finally manages to do so, this means was proven efficient.

> "Many times I almost started crying. When I managed to spur myself so that I spoke out, these bullies became a little out of countenance; how come you have the courage to defend yourself all the sudden."

Many survivors reported that their agony had not ended before school finally ended. Changing one's school was also reported as one means of coping with bullying. However, it is somewhat absurd that it is the victim who had to change the school, not the bully. It is especially unfortunate if the victim decides to quit school because of bullying.

> "I changed the school and went on with my life."

Some of the victims were able to close their minds to revenge and hatred and had forgiven their bullies hoping that they would eventually notice the bad they had done. Forgiveness is possible even if the bully did not apologize. Then, it merely represents amnesty[40].

> "…and I forgave my bullies who had so diligently bullied me for nine years… I don't carry that burden anymore."

Forgiveness follows naturally the healing process but not always. It can be difficult to forgive and therefore, forgiveness is primarily considered an act, not a feeling. Changing one's feelings can take time and may resist forgiving forever but people can also decide to forgive and thus consciously alter their emotions[40]. Forgiveness has a healing power and it can promote well-being[41].

Understanding that bullying was not the victim's fault helps in coping. As the victim understands the phenomenon in a new way, he or she is on the threshold of new direction, the process has moved on long enough and it is about to end in a situation where the victim can let go of the past. Bullying is not the victim's fault because there is not any reason justifying bullying.

> "The point is that you have to understand that the viewpoint that you had when victimized, was skewed already because of your age… Now, as an adult, I realize many, many things in bullying that I wasn't able to see when I was young. It eases a lot of the hard feelings related to those things."

Social Coping Methods

Social coping methods are means such as belonging to a group or society, adapting a certain role or task, and accepting or getting support. Basic motives of survival are social orientation and interaction[32]. The victims of bullying used their family and friends as social coping methods. According to earlier research on bullying, even a few positive peer- relationships protect a child against the long-term effects of bullying[14]. The family and friends were also perceived as the source of security.

> "No doubt, my coping was enhanced by the fact that, despite bullying, I had three friends who took care of me (although only one of them was in the same class with me). And at home, I always felt myself loved and accepted."

Social relationships also help later on when analyzing experiences. Indeed, social relationships are used for enhancing coping at every phase of the healing process. Starting one's own family was regarded as helpful in survival. One's own spouse and children provide the victim with acceptance and love that heal the wounds. In addition, a spouse's support in an intimate relationship functions as a protective measure against stress and anxiety[42].

> "But my life has been good: I have a wonderful husband, a dream job, good friends who really understand, and my firstborn will be born next summer."

Emotional Coping Methods

Anger in its various forms was strongly apparent in the victims' writings. Several writers told how they went on sustaining by the feelings of hate and the thoughts of revenge. The feeling of hate and anger can be considered to occur as the result of being the target of bullying. However, feeding the feeling of hatred may also be a means of protecting oneself against more unpleasant feelings and anxiety. Toying with the idea of revenge eases one's feelings to some extent but one should not realize the revenge. The victims also found malicious pleasure easing, especially if the victims had succeeded better in life than their bullies. Doing well in life gives strength and strengthens self-esteem.

> "…hate, hate, hate, bitterness, disappointment with your own powerlessness and that no one intervened."

> "Most of my bullies have been in jail; and I suppose their life hasn't been a bed of roses otherwise either. I'm doing quite well. So, he who laughs last laughs longest."

It is natural to want to revenge if one is being mistreated. According to the data, the thoughts of revenge could be even quite cruel:

> "…and that feeling of hate never goes away. All kinds of weird revenge plans occupy my mind quite often—how to hurt them or their family—and quite permanently. So that they could feel the same, even a little bit, the feeling that I have still in the age of 41."

Recent school shootings in Finland make an example of revenge that was actually realized. Research on massacres at school all over the world revealed that 90 % of the murderers were victims of bullying at school[43]. Bullying is not the only reason for these horrible events but it can be one factor that leads the way toward massacres. It seems that the risk is emphasized especially when the victim of bullying lacks support from school and home[44].

Hate and anger are powerful feelings that are related to the reaction phase of the crisis. It usually begins when the threat and danger situations are already over. This phase involves powerful feelings, such as hatred, guilt, fear, and sorrow. The reaction phase begins when one has to confront the situation and therefore one uses even the most primitive defense mechanism[33].

Another emotional coping method, a positive one, was positive attitude. It can be a crucial factor in the coping process[30]:

> "But maybe it's about your attitude: when you compare what your life was at some point, you won't start brooding over small issues, aches, and disappointments. They too belong to life, come and go. The most important thing is that the big picture is good."

Creative Coping Methods

The role of imagination as the thrust of people's inner life, dreams, and intuitions represent creative coping methods. Imagination is used for avoiding unpleasant facts or finding new solutions[32]. In this study, artistic hobbies and daydreaming were victims' creative coping methods. Artistic hobbies helped them to channel their anxiety in works of art and thus, their trauma had a sort of extrinsic repository in a work of art and helped to handle with bullying[45]. Creative coping methods are often used in the processing phase of trauma[34].

> "Because of bullying, I developed a strong inner world and had artistic expression as my hobby; that became the passion and strength of my life."

The power of imagination was found helpful also in the forms of daydreaming and fantasizing. The victims fantasized either about a better future or returning to time when everything was still good:

> "I dreamed my whole rough youth about the day I would be able to leave my childhood village. It helped me to cope."

> "I was happy then and have wanted to return to that time. I guess my weird dreams originate in that partly, how becoming small and fragile, physically a child, could help me to survive mentally."

Physiological Coping Methods

The physical dimension of coping is based on the thought that human behavior could be explained with stimuli, impulses, reactions, reflexes, conditioning, and reinforcement[32]. According to the data, victims of bullying had also physiological coping methods, such as sport and psychiatric medication:

> "… new hobbies, kick-boxing, and other sports—all are means of coping with it!"

> "Nowadays, I become depressed every now and then, luckily it's mild and treatable with medication"

> "I was prescribed psychopharmacon that stabilized my moods."

Spiritual Coping Methods

Two of the writers told that they survived with the help of their spiritual conviction. The other reported that spirituality helped in the healing process, too. Also in Ayalon's model, spirituality is one dimension. Belief in transcendent powers gives hopes and strength to move on[32].

> "My self-esteem has improved since that time. Jesus has helped me in difficult situations and finally I can say that I am happy."

Discussion and Conclusion

According to the results, bullying at school and coping with it is not straightforward or axiomatic. Coping is a multidimensional process and coping methods appeared somewhat overlapping. Cullberg's[33] theory of the phases of crisis is in line with the coping methods discovered in this research. Although Cullberg's theory is not the only theory that illustrates the phases of crises, it is important to know and understand what kinds of issues are related to the coping process and what one might expect. Moreover, this knowledge is important not only to victims of bullying but also to their loved ones and other helpers.

However, it is worth noticing that when long-term bullying ends, the pain and agony does not. The victim's life will be affected for a long time and he or she will need support in strengthening his or her self-esteem and position in the peer group. Without support, the victim can isolate from the society permanently even if bullying ends. Healing can be advanced by supporting the victim both at school and at home. The victim's experiences should be undermined. A child should be left alone but an adult must take the responsibility for solving the situation[46]. The earlier bullying is intervened, the better the results will be. The results of this study are also in line with findings of Ojuri's[47] who noted that coping does not mean perfect control over life but accepting the situation can also represent good coping.

Furthermore, coping is not just an upbeat success story but it can involve feelings of weakness and despair every now and then. Hopefulness, belief in change, and trustful attitude to future help moving forward. Coping includes features such as finding one's identity, liberation from guilt, and strengthening self-esteem— but on the other hand, it is holding out, acceptance, and giving up, as well[47].

Lyubomirsky[11] lists numerous studies that show relatively greater wellbeing among people who, for example, derive positive meaning from negative events and who use positive attitude (humor, spirituality, etc.) to cope with adversity and who use social comparison in adaptive ways. Also Larsen et al.[48] talk about instead of eliminating the negative, people should focus on accentuating the positive, which we understand as a positive attitude toward life events. All these strategies were evident among victims of bullying in this research.

Yet, some limitations of the results are worth addressing at this point. Collecting data from internet forums involves some problems. First, as was mentioned earlier, it is not possible to know for sure who the participants are. Second, there is no guarantee of the truthfulness of their stories. However, the forums are clearly aimed at the victims of bullying and therefore, the preliminary assumption is that people who have experienced bullying would participate in these forums. Anonymity makes it possible to write voluntarily and openly about experiences and get feedback and support from others with similar experiences. The public nature of the data also makes the researcher's task easier as there are not any difficulties in protecting the participants' anonymity: their writings are public and even the researcher does not know their identities. Third, there is the conceptual uncertainty: what is defined as bullying in these forums. In this case, we lean on the definition that emphasize that bullying is a personal experience. Therefore, people behind the pseudonyms have interpreted the mistreatment, which they have experienced, as bullying and their opinion should be respected as well.

To increase the reliability and validity of this study, excerpts from the data were added within the results. They were also supposed to convince that this data included a rich, manifold, and explicit description of bullying and coping and made a valuable contribution to the existing knowledge about the experiences of adult survivors of bullying.

Eventually, there is also one interesting point to discuss concerning the data of this research. Sharing one's story might as such represent a way of coping. It has been evidenced that people have an apparent need to share their experiences after a distressing event[10]. Writing about bullying experiences in the internet forum could be considered one way of sharing and coping with the healing process. Therefore, people who have already survived from bullying might not write in these kinds of forums. Yet, the forum is about peer support and it can be thought that people who want to support each other have at least begun their healing process.

While recognizing the problems of internet data, we want to highlight the potential that lies in the use of anonymous internet forums to discuss difficult life events, such as bullying. The potential value of translating emotional experiences into words is proved to be beneficial for coping:

"Putting upsetting experiences into words allows people to stop inhibiting their thoughts and feelings, to begin to organize their thoughts and perhaps find meaning in their traumas and to reintegrate into their social networks" [10].

Therefore, more research on the usefulness of internet forums for coping with bullying is needed and especially, how this means would help victims when at school level, children who, at this very moment, are bullied, to overcome the trauma and process the range of emotions that bullying causes.

The phenomenon of bullying is not just a problem of an individual person or groups. Bullying is a part of a larger phenomenon in our society and to which adults are partly resigned themselves. Many actions are justified by bullying: the child will not have a unique name because there is the danger that he or she will be bullied at school; parents want to buy expensive clothes, provide expensive hobbies, and gear to their children for the same reason; and so on. Parents do not want to give bullies any reason to bully their children although, when doing so, they restrict their own life assuming that they prevent bullying. Yet, it seems that for example envy, that is one of the reasons behind bullying, is not prevented this way.

What makes bullying at school extremely harmful is that a child may not necessarily understand that bullying is not his or her fault and that it cannot be reasoned in any way. The ability to understand and see the good that results from bad events is possible to develop in adulthood as many people report positive outcomes from adverse life events[49]. Focusing on the positive sides, overcoming bullying, was a conscious choice through which our aim is to take a glance at positive strategies and increase awareness of this kind of positive behavior. According to Niederhoffer and Pennebaker[10] there might be a way to use these naturally occurring processes to help individuals cope with a wide range of traumatic experiences—bullying being one of them.

However, it is worth discussing strategies that enhance positive and accepting atmosphere at schools and how they could be promoted. One of the three overarching themes of positive psychology is positive institutions[50]. Huebner et al.[51] suggest that positive schools can move away from problem-centered approaches to wellness approaches focusing on maximizing children's chances to manifest and exploit their abilities and interests recognizing that "all" students have strengths. Unquestionably, childhood may be the optimal time to promote healthy attitudes, behavior, adjustment, and prevention of problems[9] and therefore, more research on creating healthy educational environments for children is needed. For example, in Andreou's[52] study, bully/victims appeared as a distinct group in terms of their low levels of social acceptance and problem- solving ability. The most important perspective from the point of view of the present study is, especially, how to facilitate supportive teacher and peer relationships and how to maintain positive interactions among all participants at school[see also 21].

What makes the positive approach so particular? First, positive psychology is not just about non-existence of problems. Instead, it is about turning the look at well-being and factors that promote it. Dake, Price, and Telljohann[3] do a good job in reviewing the nature and extent of bullying at school, and they even introduce numerous interventions that attempt to increase students' anti-bullying attitudes. Likewise, Merrell et al.[4] point out that although anti- bullying interventions appear to be useful in increasing awareness, knowledge, and self- perceived competency in dealing with bullying, these interventions will not necessarily and dramatically

112

influence the incidence of actual bullying or positively influence the targeted outcomes.

So, bullying exists and it seems difficult to get rid of the phenomenon. The question is therefore whether the goal is too low when it is set to enhancing anti-bullying attitudes: Should it be focused on increasing wellness-promoting attitudes (acceptance, recognition, tolerance) instead to make a real difference?

References

1. Salmivalli, C. (2010). Bullying and the peer group: A review. *Aggression and Violent Behavior, 15*, 112–120.
2. Arseneault, L., Walsh, E., Trzesniewski, K., Newcombe, R., Caspi, A., & Moffitt, T. E. (2006). Bullying victimization uniquely contributes to adjustment problems in young children: A nationally representative cohort study. *Pediatrics, 118*(1), 130-138.
3. Dake, J. A., Price, J. H., & Telljohan, S. K. (2003). The nature and extent of bullying at school. *Journal of School Health, 73*(5), 173-180.
4. Merrell, K. W., Gueldner, B. A., Ross, S. W., & Isava, D. M. (2008). How effective are school bullying intervention programs? A meta-analysis of intervention research. *School Psychology Quarterly, 23*(1), 26-42.
5. Horsthemke, K. (2009). Rethinking humane education. *Ethics and Education, 4*(2), 201–214.
6. Leary, M. R., Kowalski, R. M., Smith, L., & Phillips, S. (2003). Teasing, rejection, and violence: Case studies of the school shootings. *Aggressive Behavior, 29*, 202–214.
7. Vanderbildt, D., & Augustyn, M. (2010). The effects of bullying. Pediatrics and child health. *Symposium: Special needs, 20*(7), 315-320.
8. von Marees, N., & Petermann, F. (2010). Bullying in German primary schools. *School Psychology International, 31*, 178-198.
9. Brown Kirschman, K. J., Johnson, R. J., Bender, J. A., & Roberts, M. C. (2009). Positive psychology for children and adolescents: Development, prevention, and promotion. In S. J. Lopez & C. R. Snyder (Eds.), *Oxford handbook of positive psychology* (pp. 133-147). Oxford, NY: Oxford University Press.
10. Niederhoffer, K. G., & Pennebaker, J. W. (2009). Sharing one's story: On the benefits of writing and talking about emotional experience. In S. J. Lopez & C. R. Snyder (Eds.), *Oxford handbook of positive psychology* (pp. 621-632). Oxford, NY: Oxford University Press.
11. Lyubomirsky, S. (2001). Why are some people happier than others? The role of cognitive and motivational processes in well-being. *American Psychologist, 56*(3), 239-249.
12. Chafouleas, S. M., & Bray, M. A. (2004). Introducing positive psychology: Finding a place within school psychology. *Psychology in the Schools, 41*(1), 1-6.
13. Olweus, D. (1992). *Kiusaaminen koulussa* [Bullying at school]. Helsinki: Otava.
14. Salmivalli, C. (2005). *Kaverien kanssa. Vertaissuhteet ja sosiaalinen kehitys* [With friends. Peer relationships and social development]. Jyväskylä: PS-Kustannus.
15. Pikas, A. (1990). *Irti kouluväkivallasta* [End school violence]. Imatra: Weilin+göös.
16. Harjunkoski, S.-M., & Harjunkoski, R. (1994). *Kiusanhenki lapsen kengissä. Koulukiusaaminen – haaste kasvattajalle* [A bully in a child's shoes. Bullying at school – a challenge to an educator]. Juva: Kirjapaja.
17. Unnever, J. D., & Cornell, D. G. (2004). Middle school victims of bullying: who reports being bullied? *Aggressive Behavior, 30*, 373-388.

18. Boulton, M. J., Smith, P. K., & Cowie, H. (2010). Short-term longitudinal relationships between children's peer victimization/bullying experiences and self-perceptions: evidence for reciprocity. *School Psychology International, 31,* 296-311.
19. Olweus, D. (1994). Annotation: Bullying at school: Basic facts and effects of a school based intervention program. *Journal Child Psychology and Psychiatry, 35,* 1171-1190.
20. Crick, N. R., Casa, J. F., & Ku, H.-C. (1999). Relational and physical forms of peer victimization in preschool. *Developmental Psychology, 25*(2), 376-385.
21. von Grünigen, R., Perren, S., Nagele, C., & Alsaker, F. D. (2010). Immigrant children's peer acceptance and victimization in kindergarten: The role of local language competence. *British Journal of Developmental Psychology, 28,* 679-697.
22. Shariff, S. (2009). *Confronting cyber-bullying. What schools need to know to control, misconduct and avoid legal consequences.* New York, NY: Cambridge University Press.
23. Kowalski, R. M., & Limber, S. P. (2007). Electronic bullying among middle school students. *Journal of Adolescent Health, 41,* S22-S30.
24. Perren, S., & Alsaker, F. D. (2006). Social behavior and peer relationships of victims, bully-victims, and bullies in kindergarten. *Journal of Child Psychology and Psychiatry, 47*(1), 45-57.
25. Crick, N. R., & Nelson, D. A. (2002). Relational and physical victimization within friendships: nobody told me there'd be friends like these. *Journal of Abnormal Child Psychology, 30*(6), 599-607.
26. Berger, K. (2007). Update on bullying at school: Science forgotten? *Developmental Review, 27*(1), 90-126.
27. Salmivalli, C., & Voeten, M. (2004). Connections between attitudes, group norms, and behaviour in bullying situations. *International Journal of Behavioral Development, 28*(3), 246-258.
28. Uusitalo, T. (2006). *Miten päästä yli mahdottoman* [How to cope with the impossible]. (PhD Diss., University of Lapland, Rovaniemi, Finland.)
29. Ikonen, T. (2000). *Tuhkasta uusi elämä. Selviytymisen teoreettiset ja käytännölliset lähtökohdat* [Gathering the dashes into a new life. Theoretical and practical premises for coping]. Helsinki: Helsinki University Press.
30. Furman, B. (1997). *Ei koskaan liian myöhäistä saada onnellinen lapsuus* [It's never too late to get a happy childhood]. Porvoo: WSOY.
31. Heiskanen, T. (1997). Johtolankoja selviytymistaitoihin [Leads to coping skills]. In T. Heiskanen (Ed.), *Elämäntaidon ja selviytymisen kirja* [A book of life skills and coping] (pp. 273-301). Porvoo: WSOY.
32. Ayalon, O. (1995). *Selviydyn! Yhteisön tuki ja selviytyminen* [RESCUE! Community-oriented preventive education]. (K. Absetz, Trans.). Jyväskylä: Gummerus.
33. Cullberg, J. (1991). *Tasapainon järkkyessä – psykoanalyyttinen ja sosiaalipsykiatrinen tutkielma* [Kris och utveckling, The crisis and development]. Helsinki: Otava.
34. Saari, S. (2000). *Kuin salama kirkkaalta taivaalta. Kriisit ja niistä selviytyminen* [Like a bolt from the blue. Crises and coping]. Helsinki: Otava.
35. Denzin, N. K., & Lincoln, Y. S. (2008). Introduction: The discipline and practice of qualitative research. In N. K. Denzin & Y. S. Lincoln (Eds.), *Handbook of qualitative research* (pp. 1-28). Thousand Oaks, CA: SAGE.
36. Tuomi, J., & Sarajärvi, A. (2009). *Laadullinen tutkimus ja sisällönanalyysi* [Qualitative research and content analysis]. Jyväskylä: Gummerus.
37. Laukkanen, M. (2007). *Sähköinen seksuaalisuus. Tutkimus tyttöydestä nettikeskusteluissa* [Electric sexuality. A study on girlhood in internet forums]. (PhD Diss., University of Lapland, Rovaniemi, Finland.)

114

38. Paunonen, U. (2004). <Seireeni> *huokaus*, Missä Mr. Cool? Tapaustutkimus aikuisten virtuaalisista seurusteluyhteisöistä [<Siren> *a sigh*, Where's Mr. Cool? A case study on adults' virtual dating communities]. In U. Paunonen & J. Suominen (Eds.), *Digirakkaus* [Digital love] (pp. 35-43). Turku: University of Turku.

39. Laitinen, M. (2004). *Häväistyt ruumiit, rikotut mielet* [Violated bodies, broken minds]. Tampere: Vastapaino.

40. Ojanen, M. (2007). *Positiivinen psykologia* [Positive psychology]. Helsinki: Edita.

41. Krause, W., & Ellison, C. G. (2003). Forgiveness by God, forgiveness by others and psychological wellbeing in late life. *Journal for the Scientific Study of Religion, 42*(1), 77-93.

42. Määttä, K. (2000). *Kestävä parisuhde* [Long-lasting intimate relationship]. Jyväskylä: Gummerus.

43. Verlinden, S., Hersen, M., & Thomas, J. (2000). Risk factors in school shootings. *Clinical Psychology Review, 20*(1), 3-56.

44. Punamäki, R.-L., Tirri, K., Nokelainen, P., & Marttunen, M. (2011). *Koulusurmat. Yhteiskunnalliset ja psykologiset taustat ja ehkäisy* [School massacres. Societal and psychological backgrounds and prevention]. http://www.acadsci.fi/kannanottoja/koulusurmat.pdf

45. Sarid, O., & Huss, E. (2010). Trauma and acute stress disorder: A comparison between cognitive behavioural intervention and art therapy. *The Arts in Psychotherapy, 37*, 8-12.

46. Holmberg-Kalenius, T. (2008). *Elämää koulukiusaamisen jälkeen* [Life after bullying]. Jyväskylä: Gummerus.

47. Ojuri, A. (2004). *Väkivalta naisen elämän varjona* [Violence as the shadow of a woman's life]. (PhD Diss., University of Lapland, Rovaniemi, Finland.)

48. Larsen, J. T., Hemenover, S. H., Norris, C. J., & Cacioppo, J. T. (2003). Turning the adversity to advantage: on the virtues of the coactivation of positive and negative emotions. In L. G. Aspinwall & U. M. Staudinger (Eds.), *A psychology of human strengths: Fundamental questions and future directions for a positive psychology* (pp. 211-226). Washington, D. C.: American Psychological Association.

49. Lechner, S. C., Tennen, H., & Affleck, G. (2009). Benefit-finding and growth. In S. J. Lopez & C. R. Snyder (Eds.), *Oxford handbook of positive psychology* (pp. 633-640). Oxford, NY: Oxford University Press.

50. Seligman, M. E. P., & Csikszentmihalyi, M. (2000). Positive psychology: An introduction. *American Psychologist, 60*, 410-421.

51. Huebner, E. S., Gilman, R., Reschly, A. L., & Hall, R. (2009). Positive schools. In S. J. Lopez and C. R. Snyder (Eds.), *Oxford handbook of positive psychology* (pp. 561-568). Oxford, NY: Oxford University Press.

52. Andreou, E. (2001). Bully/victim problems and their association with coping behaviour in conflictual peer interactions among school-age children. *Educational Psychology, 21*(1), 59-66.

Expertise in Health Education

Pupil Welfare Work in Finnish Schools

Teija Koskela, Kaarina Määttä and Satu Uusiautti

The guidelines for the national curriculum were revised in Finland in 2004 so that the position of pupil welfare was specified as a part of basic education[1]. Student's physical, mental, and social support was specified as the task of schools and teachers. Thus, teachers' responsibilities for students' wellbeing were expanded.

The change in teachers' work is a part of the societal change. Although the learning results are verifiably excellent at Finnish elementary schools[2], adolescents' well-being is of great concern in our society. For example, depression[3], marginalisation and exclusion[4,5], psycho-social problems[6], mental problems[7,8], and especially the increase in learning difficulties among adolescents who graduate from the comprehensive school[9] are worrying.

In Finland, compulsory education is comprehensive. Pupil welfare that protects students' well-being is not any new phenomenon at school either. However, at the moment teachers confront new challenges related to the well-being of society, school, family, and children and they consider it difficult to find methods to handle such challenges[7]. The aim of this study was to analyse how teachers realise pupil welfare tasks as a part of their job.

What is Pupil Welfare?

Defining pupil welfare is difficult because methods and concepts vary by country and school system. In Finland, the concept of pupil welfare has been connected to the promotion of physical, mental, and social well-being and prevention of the perceived threats of well-being. Pupil welfare can be seen an every student's right, and its task is to prevent exclusion[1]. It is rather similar to the concept of student care or pastoral care aiming at the development and support of the student as a person and as a social being[10]. Although wellbeing is the goal of pupil welfare, the concept of pupil welfare does not cover the whole phenomenon.

In Sweden, the methods of pupil welfare and well-being-promoting actions and the legislation that directs them are quite similar to Finland. The concept used in Sweden can be translated into student care[11,12,13]. Any further inter-Europe comparisons are harder to make because, for example, in Germany, the school system differs from the Finnish one substantially. In Germany, pupils are divided into different school levels from the fifth grade[14]; then, the heterogeneity does not affect in the same way teachers' work as it does in the comprehensive school.

In British school culture, the concept of pastoral care means action by which students' behaviour and moral are guided[15]. The methods resemble pupil welfare to a great extent. How effective pastoral care is depends on how positive an attitude the school has to the support. Integrated pastoral system refers to a school community where support has been integrated and teachers take care of pupils' wellbeing in addition to academic and disciplinary work[15,16]. Furthermore, pupil welfare is connected to the concept of 'schoolbased support'[17], which means preventative support and security, and other integrated services provided by school[18].

However, these concepts as they concentrate on individualistic support differ from the concept for pupil welfare in Finnish curricula. In the Finnish comprehensive school, teachers have relatively high responsibility for pupils' well-being. Furthermore, the services have not been described as norm-based or statutory but merely as innovative and locally provided. However, the purpose of Finnish comprehensive school is to enhance regional equality placing expectations of teachers' work for pupil welfare—and these ambitions are difficult to perceive from outside the Finnish school system[see 19].

The contentual ambiguity of pupil welfare can be dissected from the point of view of studies well-being at school. These research themes are, for example, the factors that decrease well-being at school such as the growth in school sizes[20], mental disorders, learning problems[21], and bullying at school and the risk factors related to it[22]. Disturbances in mental and social development and learning difficulties are the biggest health risk among small children and adolescents. These problems are more difficult than before[7,9,23]. On the other hand, there are factors that can promote wellbeing at school, such as the possibilities for self-fulfillment and approving and caring atmosphere[24,25]. Furthermore, it is worth remembering that even success at school does not protect students from all the factors that threaten their well-being[26]. Therefore, pupil welfare cannot be evaluated solely by looking at individual learning outcomes.

In International research, the concepts such as school attachment[20,27,28] and student–teacher bonding[20] are applied to describe well-being at school. Goodenow[29] referred to the concept of psychological membership which was later defined as school connectedness[see also 30]. Catalano, Haggerty, Oesterle, Fleming, and Hawkins[31] have regarded the concepts of school connectedness and school bonding as equal. These concepts involve both attachment which means close and emotional relationship with others and commitment which refers to engagement to school work and wish to perform well at school[31, see also 32].

A caring school is considered to enhance student's communality. In practice, communality increases students' care for others, learning motivation and problem-solving skills and the realisation of democratic values[33, see also 34]. In Finland, schools are expected to support and protect every student's holistic growth and provide everyone with equal possibilities. The Nordic idea of welfare considers comprehensive school as a wide growing environment for one phase of life and then the focus is—instead of subject-centeredness—on responsible caring and educating[see 19].

The Significance of Pupil Welfare

Well-being is constantly challenged in the school reality. Although teachers would like to focus on teaching[e.g. 7,35,36], they also need to act as communal experts and role models who compensate parenthood[37]. The change in the foci of social and societal meanings alters the expectations of teacherhood[8,38].

The Nordic welfare includes societal support as the trust in societal security systems holds the society together[39]. Society has to prevent inequality and take care of its citizens during unpredicted changes[40]. Education can intervene in the factors that cause inequality between various population groups[41]. Thus, the need for pupil welfare has increased due to all the emerging modern threats to the physical, mental, and social well-being of the population.

Pupil welfare aims at affecting not only pupils' personal well-being but also the well-being of school communities. In line with Labonte and Laverack[42], Rimpelä[43] names the most important communal aspects of health promotion capacity building at school: commitment, surveillance, and evaluations of need for support, general well-functioning practices and programs, operational structure, the stability of operations and leadership, co-operation and organisational structures. In this point of view, teachers are a part of a larger system and their ability to support and promote children's well-being develops through communication processes in a multi-professional environment.

Furthermore, families' life-management skills and ways of action have an influence on children's everyday life at school. Thus, pupil welfare at school requires cooperation with parents[19,44,45]. Societal changes reflect in families: the relationship between work and family has changed and since grandparents and other relatives work too, less support is received from them than before. Furthermore, parents' mental problems and substance abuse, unemployment or excessive stress at work cause complex problems in families. The need for multi-professional pupil welfare becomes especially pronounced when a child is taken into custody[46]. In all, the role of pupil welfare has become more and more important as it has to solve the problems in parenthood as well[23,47].

Problems in individual students' well-being increase the need for pupil welfare the most directly. Estimations about the number of children who need support vary. According to STAKES[23], about every third student has problems that require further examination or attention if also difficulties in communication and learning are taken into account. Behavioural and emotional problems have increased and problems are more serious than before[7,21].

Methods

The role of school in promoting students' well-being is, therefore, salient: school can support and direct the development process in a positive direction[43]. Teachers' work changes along these expectations and they are expected to have knowledge and skills to meet the new expectations[48,49]. The aim of this study was to study the state and realisation of pupil welfare at schools through perceptions of the teachers' who work with pupil welfare. Teachers were asked to discuss this work task and the success of pupil welfare. The following questions were set for this study:

(1) How did teachers' perceptions of pupil welfare work differ?

(2) What kind of overall picture of pupil welfare in comprehensive education as a part of teachers' work can be drawn according to the teachers' perceptions?

The first research question is dissected through the data. These findings are then compiled and further analysed. This compilation is presented in the Conclusions Section.

Fifteen teachers (14 women and 1 man) from eight municipalities in the province of Lapland, in northern Finland were interviewed. The teachers worked as classroom teachers, subject teachers, student counsellors, principals, or special teachers in Finnish comprehensive education (grades 1–9). Some teachers' work was a combination of the above-mentioned positions and, thus, their job descriptions were quite wideranging which is rather usual in sparsely populated areas like northern Finland. In this article, the participants are commonly called teachers.

This was a qualitative study with the aim of providing the participants with the role of empowered respondent[50], and the participants were recruited by a so-called snow-ball sampling[51]. The starting point of the snow-ball sampling was an in-service training period of pupil welfare. The participants in the training were asked to give their contact information if they were willing to participate in the preliminary interviews. The research data were collected through qualitative and voluntary interviews in the fall 2006. The final data comprised 15 interviews that varied from 64 minutes to 2 hours and 27 minutes.

It is a challenge if an interviewee is not familiar with the theme of the interview or if he or she has not even thought about it, interview can produce merely assumptions than actual perceptions or experiences. To avoid this serious problem, all interviewees got a letter before the actual interview. It consisted of a short description of the research and five different starting questions. The interviewees could select the starting question but they were also offered the possibility to start the interview with some other important issue. Furthermore, the participants could decide what and how they wanted to say about their own work with pupil welfare.

The research method was phenomenography where interview is quite a common data collection method[52]. This kind of profound interview method enables the participants to produce meanings through reflective dialogue[53]. In this research, the interviewees were allowed to discuss their perceptions of pupil welfare as extensively as possible without any strict or pre-determined questions.

The data were analysed through categorisation. The basic unit was a description of an experience or insight. The shortest excerpts that functioned as analysing units could be only few words long while the longest included a description of processes that belong to pupil welfare. The contents of these basic units mattered and therefore, bringing out the individual who expressed an experience or insight was not considered important. The categorisation had three main stages. First, the data were organised by the words or concepts used in the interviews resulting in dozens of categories. In the second categorisation round, the data were arranged by a revised categorisation structure with more specific, yet unstructured categories such as interaction, multiprofessionalism, and student-specific processes. In the third categorisation, the data were finally arranged within carefully defined categories with sub-categories[e.g. 54] representing higher level of abstraction.

Results

Teachers' perceptions of pupil welfare could be divided into two fundamental categories: commitment to pupil welfare work and trust in work environment. It is worth pointing out that the purpose was not to categorise teachers themselves based on their commitment but their perceptions that had emerged in some particular work situations within particular work contexts.

Differences in Teachers' Commitment to Pupil Welfare Work

Commitment to work on pupil welfare means directing one's motivation in welfare work. Commitment appears as interest in and willingness to spend time with welfare work and the ability to make oneself vulnerable to insecurity or criticism when intervening in sensitive welfare-related matters. Furthermore, commitment seemed to include desire to develop pupil welfare at school. According to the participants, commitment was manifested by following the agreements, plans of action and schedules, and willingness to change the individual or group's way of action to meet the needs of pupil welfare work. Pupil welfare work also included teachers' activity in following processes, taking care of the progress, and acquiring required resources. According to teachers' perceptions, commitment to pupil welfare work covers both individual and communal levels. For example, a good work community was considered supportive and encouraging also in times of failure or other difficult situations.

Strong commitment to pupil welfare work means that one has to arrange time for it and be prepared to negotiate and willing to look for options for changing one's ownway of action. Furthermore, commitment was considered the ability to notice when there was need for taking action and following them through even if that required overwork:

> . . . if you take care of something properly, it'll take lots of time.

> I do think that if you worry about something you have to find the time to take care of it.

> Some things are not necessarily [taken care of] because some people have the principle that they don't do overtime because you don't get paid. But I don't know about that then...

Some of the teachers thought that they were committed to pupil welfare work. But it was not considered something that every teacher would do:

> It is not obligatory. Basically, according to the law, we have to do pupil welfare work but it is left to every teacher to decide how dutifully their do it.

Teachers said that because of hurry and lack of time pupil welfare work was sometimes passed over. Teacher did not have resources to interfere with everything:

> Yeah, that; or should I just pass it. No. I'm not interested in this at the moment, although it seems like time to intervene but I don't bother. I'll avoid the trouble if I don't address it at all.

Therefore, weak commitment appeared as trouble finding time for pupil welfare work, unwillingness to participate in negotiations or take actions. Weak commitment was explained by outer reason and manifested by passiveness in negotiations, questioning others' action and having prejudiced, or unwillingness to engage in measures of action that would change one's own way of action.

Differences in Teachers' Trust in Work Environment

In this study, trust in the work environment illustrates the relationship between a teacher who is committed to pupil welfare work and his or her environment. It includes the existence of supportive structures and the teacher's notion on his or her possibilities to make use of them. The teachers defined trust as the predictability of people and services related to pupil welfare and the possibility to interpret instructions, norms, and practices in a way that supports it. Trust was manifested as available information and opportunities to share experiences.

According to the data, teachers' experiences of sharing information and experiences differed. Some mentioned that the flow of information within one school building or organisation had proven challenging or even impossible. Similarly, even if there were quite systematic plans for distributing information, the channels still did not work.

The teachers also reported different kinds of needs to get information about pupils: some considered thorough communication with others salient, whereas others questioned the need for sharing detailed pupil-specific information:

> .. we had the very first teachers' meeting and there they told to everyone that this pupil had this kind of difficulty...So I was just thinking that what is the use of sharing this information with everyone.

Well not really. Actually, I'm not allowed to share this information. At least, so I have understood.

In a work environment where strong commitment to pupil welfare work was present, many contacts between multi-professional pupil welfare personnel occurred and cooperation was considered efficient. For example, the teachers regarded healthcare services reachable and healthcare nurses were seen as co-workers with whom teachers could share the responsibility for students' well-being. However, in small schools in sparsely populated areas, the services are scarce. Therefore, the teachers were also concerned about the realisation of pupils' legal protection.

...we would really make use of the services of a psychologist or a social worker or a doctor or all of them. So we would benefit from them but we don't have the possibility because there aren't especially many; I guess one psychologist or pediatrician working at the moment and not a specific school doctor; so that health clinic doctors visit and...

...you can't even think that they would start such a process here for some student that he/ she would put on a six-week follow-up study in The Central Hospital of Lapland.

According to the teachers, pupil welfare work also required social skills, interaction skills, persistency, negotiating skills, and methodicalness not only when talking about welfare issues with school personnel but with parents as well:

And pupil welfare demands persistency... perseverance, methodicalness, and that persistency.

Not only an individual teacher needs these features but also the whole pupil welfare team. Lack of trust was perceived by the teachers as a reason why pupil welfare work was not shared but carried out alone, working by oneself. In an environment of weak trust, things happen unexpectedly and actors are not aware of each other's activities. The teachers described their mutual distrust as ignorance or renouncement of agreed practices. The division of labour in pupil welfare work was considered burdensome to those who were committed to it. Lack of support exhausted teachers:

I think that pupil welfare should be everybody's business so that it concerns everyone who works here. I mean if you think that pupils work here and so do teachers and our cleaners, cookers, caretakers, it concerns everyone's well-being...

Because this work requires interaction and if a teacher is to interact well with pupils, he or she has to feel great at the work place.

Therefore, the interpretation of well-being may also differ among personnel. In addition, the service structure is random and the profitability of pupil welfare

124

work can be questioned. Plenty of resources were used on reducing the resistance and building trust especially in the profitability of pupil welfare work. Trust described a teacher's own relationship with other's action and doing things together.

Conclusion: The Typology of Pupil Welfare Work

Based on the teachers' perceptions, an overall picture of pupil welfare work in comprehensive education as a part of teachers' work was drawn. The teachers' commitment to pupil welfare work varied between strong and weak but the same kind of variation could be interpreted from their trust in the work environment. Based on these two dimensions, pupil welfare work can be presented in an overall model where it is divided into four types: backlogging, disintegrated, sectoral, or participatory (see Figure 1).

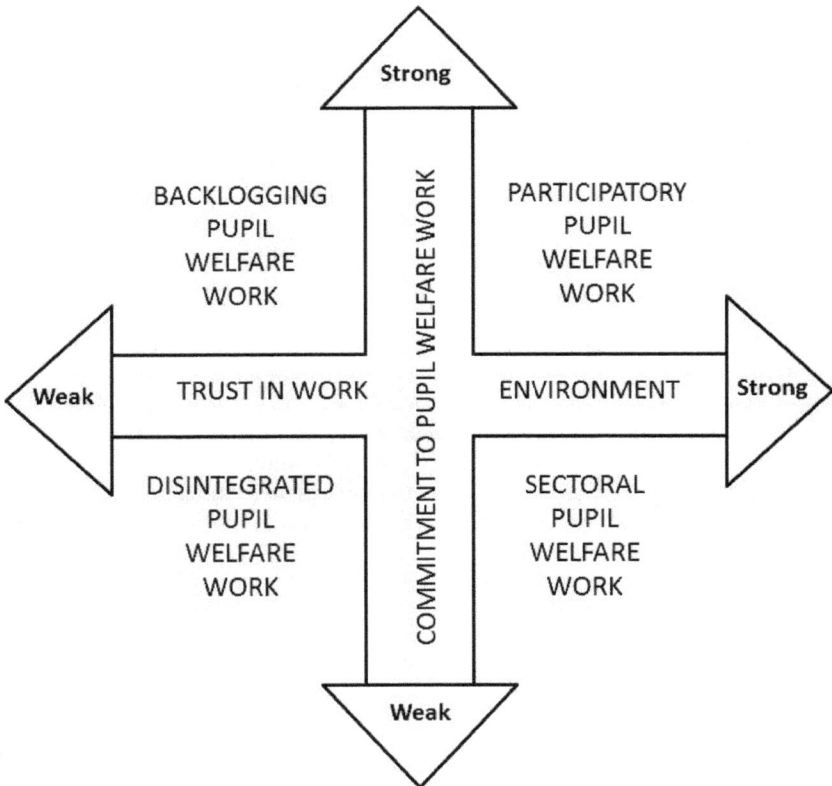

Figure 1. The typology of pupil welfare work[19, p.230].

In backlogging pupil welfare work, teachers face excessive strain when trying to take care of multi-professional pupil welfare work alone and committedly. There are not any supporting structures or if there are, they cannot be applied for pupil welfare work. Teachers find it difficult to find a partner to work with in pupil welfare. Teachers have to or want to do pupil welfare work specifically by themselves.

When disintegrated, pupil welfare work is ignored by every quarter. The supporting services for pupil welfare are not easily reachable. The possibilities for cooperation are regarded as minimal, and the interest in the everyday life at school does not focus on the pupil welfare matters. It is difficult to find anyone who takes the responsibility. Pupil welfare work is carried out neither alone nor together.

Sectoral pupil welfare work offers a good work environment and related services. However, following and summing up things may remain insignificant. Pupil welfare work may outstrip its primary target, the pupil, and the cooperation related to pupil welfare work is in danger of turning into inefficient or self-sufficient. Pupil welfare work is outsourced to others. The supporting processes fall by the wayside, remain unconnected to each other, or inefficient. The mutual advantages and profits of the adults who participate in pupil welfare processes, such as social interaction, may outrun pupils' needs. The striving for consensus becomes more important than the evaluation and pupil welfare work starts to repeat certain pupil welfare activities purposelessly.

In participatory pupil welfare work, the school structures and working environments support and appreciate pupil welfare. The reliability and predictability of the service structure and the commitment of the school community result in the focused and developing realisation of pupil welfare work. The measures of support are followed and evaluated. The various parties in pupil welfare work are capable of having dialogic conversation and thus, discussing the challenging situations becomes easier. Pupil welfare work is efficient and functional and carried out by individuals and together.

Discussion

Limitations

Qualitative research can be evaluated through the relationship and correspondence between the results and the original data[55]. In this research, the categories and the structures of variations are interpretations that are based on the research data. The interpretation and conceptualisation rest on the data and the expressions the teachers used. The citations from the interviews presented in this article are to convince readers of the reliability of the research and to bring out the participants' voices; which is also typical of phenomenographic research.

However, the results of this research are based on time- and place-bound interviews and they cannot be generalised as such. In addition to the interview situations, the data involve time-bound emphases and limitations. For example, immigrants were not mentioned at all in the data as there is hardly any in these municipalities of northern Finland where the participants of this study worked. Therefore, the generalisability of the framework produced in this research can be questioned nor is generalisation even the goal but reporting teachers' perceptions and finding ways to advance pupil welfare work in schools through teachers' hands-on experiences.

Implications for School Health

The common debate about children's and adolescents' indisposition has not managed to guarantee regionally, structurally, and qualitatively comprehensive supply of pupil welfare services. The incoherence of the pupil welfare concepts is evident in the data of this research as well. In addition, the model introduced in this article shows that the success of pupil welfare work in schools is not just about teachers' willingness (or unwillingness) to commit to it but also the support (or lack of support) provided by the work environment. The study shows that the concept of pupil welfare should be discussed and defined together with professionals who work with pupil welfare issues to enhance the multi-professional co-operation in schools. Similarly, various regional conditions should be taken into account. This study was conducted in Finnish Lapland where the conditions differ considerably from the conditions in southern Finland.

Teachers are at the central position as they work with children at school every day. Teachers have great possibilities to do welfare work as long as their proficiency and working conditions are taken care of. It has been shown that if workers have an opportunity to develop and acquire required skills so that it does not harm the completion of their basic work tasks, they will have a positive attitude toward changes and new work tasks[see e.g., 56,57,58]. Furthermore, the multi-professional nature and communality in pupil welfare demand to dismantle the myth of working alone in a teacher's professional[59] already during teacher education[e.g., 60].

On the other hand, the economic issues related to pupil welfare work should be brought out as well. Efficient pupil welfare work necessitates new conditions to teachers' working hours and payment. If pupil welfare work was considered as a fixed part of teachers' work, it should be defined distinctively in teachers' working hours.

However, the problem cannot be solved just by raising teachers' wages: it will not remove their stress but more unambiguous definition for working hours, more extensive supportive structures, and new activities and renewal of school structures are needed. A teacher who is committed to pupil welfare work has to be an expert of child development.

However, it would worth contemplating that in the modern world, pupil welfare work does not rest solely on financial or structural premises. The values and appreciations are changing and more and more attention is paid on positive development and success despite of just preventing dysfunctions[61,62,63]—and it concerns the school as well.

The fundamental idea and focus on human well-being could be defining principle also when arranging pupil welfare work: teaching the various professionals who work with pupils caring attitude and showing the positive power of love[49,64,65,66,67]. From this point of view, also teacher education can be seen differently. If the ability of being a caring adult and educator is required of a teacher, can we expect that these qualifications develop in teachers naturally and together with substance knowledge? The whole debate regarding pupil welfare work should be included as a part of discussion about the responsibilities of school and about the change in the modern teacherhood.

References

1. *Peruskoulun opetussuunnitelman perusteet 1994* [The national core curriculum 1994]. Helsinki: Finnish National Board of Education.
2. Kupiainen, S., Hautamäki, J., & Karjalainen, T. (2009). *The Finnish education system and PISA*. Helsinki: Ministry of Education.
3. Bhatia, S. K., & Bhatia, S. C. (2007). Childhood and adolescent depression. *American Family Physician, 75*(1), 73–80.
4. Martin, M. (2005). The causes and nature of bullying and social exclusion in schools. *Education Journal, 86*, 28–30.
5. Messiou, K. (2006). Conversations with children: Making sense of marginalisation on primary school settings. *European Journal of Special Needs Education, 21*(1), 39–54.
6. Hjern, A., Alfven, G., & Östberg, V. (2008). School stressors, psychological complaints and sychosomatic pain. *Acta Paediatrica, 97*, 112–117.
7. Webb, R., Vuillamy, G., Hämäläinen, S., Sarja, A., Kimonen, E., & Nevalainen, R. (2004). Pressures, rewards and teacher retention: A comparative study of primary teaching in England and Finland. *Scandinavian Journal of Educational Research, 48*(2), 169–188.
8. Williams, J. H., Horvath, V. E., Wei, H., Van Dorn, R. A., & Johnson-Reid, M. (2007). Teachers' perspectives of children's mental health service needs in urban elementary schools. *Children & Schools, 29*(2), 95–107.
9. Pietikäinen, M., & Ala-Laurila, E. (2002). Oppilashuoltotyö [Pupil welfare work]. In M. Rimpelä, A.-M. Rogoff, J. Kuusela, & H. Peltonen (Eds.), *Hyvinvoinnin ja terveyden edistäminen peruskouluissa. Perusraportti kyselystä 7.-9. vuosiluokkien kouluille* [Promotion of wellbeing and health at comprehensive schools. The basic report about the inquiry for the schools with 7–9 grades] (pp. 40–48). Helsinki: National Board of Education.
10. Best, R. (2002). *Pastoral care & personal–social education*. Roehampton: University of Surrey.
11. Andersson, G., Pösö, T., Väisänen, E., & Wallin, A. (2002). School social work in Finland and other Nordic countries: Cooperative professionalism in schools. In M. Huxtable & E. Blyth (Eds.), *School social work worldwide* (pp. 77–92). Washington, DC: National Association of Social Workers.

128

12. Backlund, A. (2007). *Elevvard I grundskolan – Resurser, organisering och praktik* [Student care in comprehensive school – resources, organizing and practice] (Report of Social Work, No. 121). Stockholm: University of Stockholm.

13. Näsman, E., & Lunden, A. (1980). *Elevvard – Till vems bra?* [Student care – For whose best?]. Stockholm: Prisma.

14. Werning, R., Löser, J., & Urban, M. (2008). Cultural and social diversity. An analysis of minority groups in German schools. *The Journal of Special Education, 42*(1), 47–54.

15. Hamblin, D. (1979). *The teacher and pastoral care.* Oxford: Basil Blackwell.

16. Nelson, E., & White, D. (2001). Pastoral care for children of cancer patients. *Pastoral Care in Education: An International Journal of Personal, Social and Emotional Development, 19*(3), 2–9.

17. Sugai, G. (2003). Commentary, establishing efficient and durable systems of school-based support. *School Psychology Review, 32*(4), 530–535.

18. Forbes, J. (2006). Types of social capital: Tools to explore service integration? *International Journal of Inclusive Education, 10*(6), 565–580.

19. Koskela, T. (2009). *Perusopetuksen oppilashuolto Lapissa opettajien käsitysten mukaan* [Teachers' conceptions of pupil welfare in basic education in Lapland] (PhD Diss., University of Lapland, Rovaniemi, Finland.)

20. Crosnoe, R., Johnson, M. K., & Elder, G. H. (2004). School size and the interpersonal side of education: An examination of race/ethnicity and organizational context. *Social Science Quarterly, 85*(5), 1259–1274.

21. Pönkkö, M.-L. (2005). *Erityisoppilaan psykiatrinen hoitoketju* [The Psychiatric treatment process of a special student] (PhD Diss., University of Oulu, Oulu, Finland.)

22. Nordhagen, R., Nielsen, A., Stigum, H., & Köhler, L. (2005). Parental reported bullying among Nordic children: A population-based study. *Child: Care, Health & Development, 31*(6), 639–701.

23. STAKES. (2008). *Erityisopetukseen siirretyt peruskoulun oppilaat lääneittäin ja kunnittain syksyllä 2007* [Comprehensive school pupils who were transformed in special education by provinces and municipalities in the fall 2007]. http://www.stat.fi(erop/2007/erop_2007_2008-06-10_tau_007.html

24. Konu, A. (2002). *Oppilaiden hyvinvointi koulussa* [Students' well-being at school] (PhD Diss., University of Tampere, Tampere, Finland.)

25. Libbey, H. P. (2004). Measuring student relationship to school: Attachment, bonding, connectedness and engagement. *Journal of School Health, 74*(7), 274–283.

26. Gerard, J. M., & Buehler, C. (2004). Cumulative environmental risk and youth maladjustment: The role of youth attributes. *Child Development, 75*(6), 1832–1849.

27. Henry, K., & Slater, M. (2007). The contextual effect of school attachment on young adolescents' alcohol use. *Journal on School Health, 77*(2), 67–74.

28. Hill, L., & Werner, N. E. (2006). Affiliative motivation, school attachment and aggression in school. *Psychology in the Schools, 43*(2), 231–246.

29. Goodenow, C. (1993). The psychological sense of school membership among adolescents: Scale development and educational correlates. *Psychology in the Schools, 30*, 79–90.

30. Shochet, I. M., Dadds, M. R., Ham, D., & Montague, R. (2006). School connectedness is an underemphasized parameter in adolescent mental health: Results of a community prediction study. *Journal of Clinical Child and Adolescent Psychology, 35*(2), 170–179.

31. Catalano, R. F., Haggerty, K. P., Oesterle, S., Fleming, C. B., & Hawkins, J. D. (2004). The importance on bonding to school for healthy development: Findings from the social development research group. *Journal on School Health, 47*(7), 252–261.

129

32.	Wilson, D. (2004). The interface of school climate and school connectedness and relationships with aggression and victimization. *Journal on School Health, 47*(7), 293–299.
33.	Battistich, V., Solomon, D., Watson, M., & Scaps, E. (1997). Caring school communities. *Educational Psychologist, 32*(3), 137–151.
34.	Noddings, N. (2005). *The challenge to care in schools. An alternative approach to education* (2nd ed.). New York, NY: Columbia University.
35.	Bryck, A., & Scheiner, B. (2003). Trust in schools: A core resource for school reform Association for supervision and curriculum development. *Educational Leadership, 60*(6), 40–44.
36.	Pedder, D., & McIntyre, D. (2006). Pupil consultation: The importance of social capital. *Educational Review, 58*(2), 144–157.
37.	UNESCO, & OECD. (2001). *Teachers for tomorrow's schools. Analysis of the world education indicators.* Paris: UNESCO Publishing.
38.	Helterbran, V. R. (2008). Professionalism: Teachers taking the reins. *The Clearing House, 81*(3), 123–127.
39.	Lehto, M. (2003). Sosiaalipolitiikka ja hyvinvointivaltion tulevaisuus [Social Policy and the future of the welfare state]. In M. Laitinen & A. Pohjola (Eds.), *Sosiaalisen vaihtuvat vastuut* [The changing responsibility of the social] (pp. 163–194). Helsinki: Dialogia.
40.	McClelland, A. (2002). Mutual obligation and the welfare responsibilities of government. *Harvard Educational Review, 62*(3), 279–300.
41.	Koivusilta, L., & Rimpelä, A. (2002). Koulu terveydellisen tasa-arvon edistäjänä [School as a promotor of healh equality]. In I. Kangas, I. Keskimäki, S. Koskinen, K. Manderbacka, E. Lahelma, R. Prättälä, & M. Sihto (Eds.), *Kohti terveyden tasa-arvoa* [Toward the equality in health] (pp. 221–235). Helsinki: Edita.
42.	Labonte, R., & Laverack, G. (2001). Capacity building in health promotion, Part 2: Whose use? And with what measures? *Critical Public Health, 11*(2), 129–138.
43.	Rimpelä, M. (2007). Terveydenedistämisaktiivisuus [Activeness in health promotion]. In M. Rimpelä, A.-M. Rogoff, J. Kuusela, & H. Peltonen (Eds.), *Hyvinvoinnin ja terveyden edistäminen peruskouluissa. Perusraportti kyselystä 7.-9. vuosiluokkien kouluille* [Promotion of wellbeing and health at comprehensive schools. The basic report about the inquiry for the schools with 7–9 grades] (pp. 17–23). Helsinki: National Board of Education.
44.	Huxtable, M., & Blyth, E. (2002). Introduction. In M. Huxtable & E. Blyth (Eds.), *School social work worldwide* (pp. 1–14). Washington, DC: National Association of Social Workers.
45.	Posch, P. (2000). Community, school change, and strategic networking. In H. Altrichter & J. Elliot (Eds.), *Images of educational change* (pp. 55–65). Buckingham: Open University Press.
46.	Coulling, N. (2000). Definitions of successful education for the looked after child: A multiagency perspective. *Support for Learning, 15*(1), 30–35.
47.	Coleman, J. S. (1988). Social capital in the creation of human capital. *American Journal of Sociology, 94*, S95–S120.
48.	van Horn, J. E., Schaufeli, W. B., & Enzmann, D. (1999). Teacher burnout and lack of reciprocity. *Journal of Applied Social Psychology, 29*, 81–108.
49.	Määttä, K., & Uusiautti, S. (2011). Pedagogical love and good teacherhood. *Education, 17*(2). http://ineducation.ca/article/pedagogical-love-and-good-teacherhood
50.	Tierney, W. G., & Dilley, P. (2001). Interviewing in education. In J.F. Gubrium & J.A. Holstein (Eds.), *Handbook of interview research* (pp. 453–471). Thousand Oaks, CA: Sage.
51.	Warren, C. A. B. (2001). Qualitative interviewing. In J.F. Gubrium & J.A. Holstein (Eds.), *Handbook of interview research* (pp. 83–101). Thousand Oaks, CA: Sage.

130

52. Francis, H. (1993). Advancing phenomenography: Questions of method. *Nordisk Pedagogik, 13*, 68–75.
53. Niikko, A. (2003). *Fenomenografia kasvatustieteellisessä tutkimuksessa* [Phenomengraphy in educational research]. Joensuu: University of Joensuu.
54. Bowden, J. (2005). Reflections on the phenomenographic team research process. In J. Bowden & P. Green (Eds.), *Doing developmental phenomengraphy* (pp. 11–31). Melbourne: RMIT University Press.
55. Guba, E. G., & Lincoln, Y. S. (2005). Paradigmatic controversies, contradictions, and emerging confluences. In N. K. Denzin & Y. S. Lincoln (Eds.), *The Sage handbook of qualitative research* (pp. 191–216). Thousand Oaks, CA: Sage.
56. Lehto, A.-M., Sutela, H., & Miettinen, A. (Eds.). (2006). *Kaikilla mausteilla. Artikkeleita työolotutkimuksesta* [With all spices. Articles research at working conditions]. Helsinki: STAKES.
57. Mäkikangas, A. (2007). *Personality, well-being and job-resources. From negative paradigm towards positive psychology.* Jyväskylä: University of Jyväskylä.
58. Uusiautti, S., & Määttä, K. (2010). What kind of employees become awarded of the Year in Finland? *Enterprise and Work Innovation Studies, 6*, 53–73.
59. Parker, M. A., Ndoye, A., & Imig, S. R. (2009). Keeping our teachers! Investigating mentoring practices to support and retain novice educators. *Mentoring & Tutoring: Partnership in Learning, 17*(4), 329–341.
60. Jakku Sihvonen, R. (Ed.). (2005). *Uudenlaisia maistereita. Kasvatusalan koulutuksen kehittämislinjoja* [New kinds of masters: Developmental guidelines of education of the educational sciences]. Jyväskylä: PS-kustannus.
61. Carruthers, C., & Hood, C.D. (2005). The power of positive psychology. *Parks & Recreation, 40*(10), 30–37.
62. Määttä, K. (Ed.) (2007). *Helposti särkyvää. Nuoren kasvun turvaaminen* [Fragile – securing youngsters' growth]. Helsinki: Kirjapaja.
63. Magnusson, D., & Mahoney, J. L. (2006). Holistinen lähestymistapa myönteisen kehityksen tutkimuksessa [A holistic perspective on the positive development research]. In L. G. Aspinwall & U. M. Staudinger (Eds.), *Ihmisen vahvuuksien psykologia* [A psychology of human strengths] (pp. 232–250). Helsinki: Edita.
64. Määttä, K., & Uusiautti, S. (2012). How do the Finnish family policy and early education system support the well-being, happiness, and success of families and children? *Early Child Development and Care, 182*(3–4), 291–298.
65. van Manen, M. (1991). *The tact of teaching: The meaning of pedagogical thoughtfulness.* London: Althouse Press.
66. Paldanius, A., & Määttä, K. (2011). What are students' views of (loving) caring in nursing education in Finland? *International Journal of Caring Sciences, 4*(2), 81–89.
67. Skinnari, S. (2004). *Pedagoginen rakkaus. Kasvattaja elämän tarkoituksen ja ihmisen arvoituksen äärellä* [Pedagogical love. Educator by the meaning of life and riddle of human being]. Jyväskylä: PS-Kustannus.

How to Promote the Healthy Development of Human Resources in Children and Youth?

Satu Uusiautti and Kaarina Määttä

Jungle of Concepts: The Connection between Human Resources and Positive Development and Health

Every human being's life is filled with promises and chances, and strengths and positive resources do not belong to just certain people. Happiness and satisfaction must be understood as the outcome of an interaction process between individual characteristics and aspirations on the one side, and social relations and macro-social structures on the other side[1]. It seems that endeavors to increase happiness and well-being have become increasingly more popular in educational settings[2]. Positive psychology offers a suitable theoretical basis for conceptualizing and planning such interventions[3,4]. One basic idea is that well-being is not only valuable because it feels good but also because it has beneficial effects not only for the individual[see 5] but also for society[6].

Luthans et al.[7,8] emphasize that knowing "who I am" is equally important as "what I know" and "who I know". The researchers call it positive psychological capital and claim that by focusing on personal strengths and good qualities, people's confidence, hope, optimism, and resilience can be developed. Psychological capital has been defined as "an individual's positive psychological state of development and is characterized by: (1) having confidence (self-efficacy) to take on and put in the necessary effort to succeed at challenging tasks; (2) making a positive attribution (optimism) about succeeding now and in the future; (3) persevering toward goals and, when necessary, redirecting paths to goals (hope) in order to succeed; and (4) when beset by problems and adversity, sustaining and bouncing back and even beyond (resilience) to attain success"[8, p.542]. A human being is an entity: Psychological capital also has a positive influence on physical health[e.g.,9], whereas mental health and human capital problems tend to co-occur with physical health problems and substance dependence[e.g., 10]. Indeed, Avey et al.[11] have pointed out that within the behavioral sciences, there has been a specific focus on the importance of well-being, both physical and mental health, in affecting success in many life domains.

But what are those strong internal personal resources or individual and why do they matter? How they could be harnessed for the use of education and eventually to benefit children's and youngsters' positive development? In this article, we will provide a review of the factors that are shown to be connected with positive mental and social health. The impact of positive emotions, relationships, and life events in mental health is indisputable[e.g., 12]. However, many studies have actually shown that such factors also maintain or improve physical health, too, J. R. Edwards and C. L. Cooper[13] being among the first researchers suggesting the possibility of positive emotions influencing to also physical health. Their research was based on stress studies presenting the concept of eustress. After that, the connection between positive states and both mental and physical health has become established. For example, Taylor et al.[14] concluded that "psychological beliefs such as meaning, control, and optimism act as resources, which may not only preserve mental health in the context of traumatic or life-threatening events but be protective of physical health as well"[14, p. 99].

As the introduction shows, the recent (positive) psychological research has introduced various viewpoints to the connection between human flourishing and healthy development[see also 15]. Indeed, there are numerous ways of approaching the phenomenon. One of the most famous and recognized attempts is probably Diener's theory of subjective well-being. Diener et al.[16] conceptualized psychological or subjective well-being as a broad construct, encompassing four specific and distinct components including (a) pleasant affect or positive well-being (e.g., joy, elation, happiness, mental health), (b) unpleasant affect or psychological distress (e.g., guilt, shame, sadness, anxiety, worry, anger, stress, depression), (c) life satisfaction (a global evaluation of one's life), and (d) domain or situation satisfaction (e.g., work, family, leisure, health, finances, self)[see also 17].

While Diener's theory focuses on merely to the state people pursue, another way of analyzing favorable outcomes is to focus on the individual and his or her possibilities to develop and find fulfillment. This means that it is reasonable to pay attention to human strengths. Recently, more and more attention has been paid on studying human virtues or strengths[18] and even detailed classifications of human strengths are available[see 19]. Now, research on human weaknesses has to compete with strong interest in human abilities, healthy aptitudes, and virtues[20].

The concept of human strengths can be considered as contextually dynamic because the function of a specific behavior depends on its context and its outcome. In addition, contexts are dynamic and change during an individual's life span. The concept of human strengths is also norm-dependent because the fundamental features of a society involve common knowledge about appropriate and appreciated behavior[21]. Magnusson and Mahoney[18] introduce two perspectives on the use and purpose of human strengths. Synchronic perspective tries to explain an individual's behavior based on the psychological and biological orientations at a certain moment. Whereas diachronic point of view is interested in those developmental processes that have led to the prevailing behavior.

Our especial point of view is to consider the promotion and use of strengths as issues that teachers and educators need to address. Along with the goals of basic education[22], teachers' action is to promote high-quality learning but also pupils' personal growth and well-being. It necessary to perceive what the various dimensions of human resources and their connection to health are.

Our viewpoints strongly lean on the idea of positive influence and positive education as the promoters of health and well-being. According to Seligman et al.[23, p. 295], "well-being should be taught in school on three grounds: as an antidote to depression, as a vehicle for increasing life satisfaction, and as an aid to better learning and more creative thinking." Furthermore, Huebner et al.[24, pp.565-566] have defined the features of positive schools. They emphasize that today's positive schools appreciate the importance of subjective well-being, treat students as individuals, and facilitate supportive teacher and peer relationships. Thus, positive schools can promote healthy development in various ways and at various levels. Next, we will discuss this in more detail.

What is the Basis of Positive, Healthy Development?

Positive psychology, which deals with such issues as well-being, happiness, the quality of life and positive feelings, has been concerned with investigating positive characteristics and feelings as well as the institutions that facilitate the discovery of positive feelings and strengths[25,26]. We will introduce some key aspects that we want to emphasize when defining the basic features of positive development. We distinguish four dimensions that each contribute to the overall sense of well-being and that educators should pay attention to when aiming at supporting children's and youngsters' healthy life-styles and balanced development, also later in life [see also 27,28].

Positive Feelings

Joy and contentment, optimism, being appreciated and feeling of security create positive mood, fundamental positive attitude that affect positively well-being at work in numerous ways. Positive emotions support problem-solving skills and the ability to act in an innovative way and thus increase human well-being. The importance and potential of this may seem surprising as the feelings of happiness are so simple and common in nature[29]. Another reason why beneficial effects of positive feelings may seem surprising is that people do not usually look for reasons or explanations when things go well.

However, experience has already shown that the healthier and more satisfied people are the better they function[30]. It is notable that positive emotional states are believed to be associated with good social relationships[30] because optimistic, joyful and self-confident people with a sense of personal control may have more social support[31], may have better social attractiveness[e.g.,32] and social skills and self-efficacy[e.g., 33].

Good Social Relationships

People live in the network of human relationships their whole life. Many people find the meaning of life within the framework of relationships. For example, Berscheid[34] claims that understanding human behavior has suffered because of forgetting this fact. However, most of the behavior takes place in the context of human relationships.

Everyone needs intimate relationships which provide appreciation, support, recreation, and protection. In school context, Pyhältö, Soini, and Pietarinen's[22] study showed that the possibility and ability to use the social resources of the school environment (especially when combined with a sense of active learning agency) could protect from for example experiences of anxiety and emotional distress. Likewise, a large Russian study showed that social capital increases physical and emotional health more than human capital, and together they can easily raise an individual's self-reported health to good health[35].

Sufficient Self-Regulation and Self-Appreciation

In Ancient Greece, lack of will and determination was considered the reason for unsatisfactory life and thus, they regarded the strength of character, self-discipline, and ability to control impulses as the prerequisite of a good life. Any great plans or long-term goals cannot be achieved without self-appreciation, perseverance, commitment and the ability to control and channel impulses.

Optimism has a clear connection to success because among other things, it involves the ability to set reasonable goals, to achieve these goals, and to use efficient learning strategies. According to Carver and Scheier[36], optimistic people achieve their goals because they organize their actions in an intellectual way. Proactive attitude (as opposed to reactive)[see 37,38] also represents such cognitive resources. Proactive people can change their behavior, see things from a different light, make choices, and know what they want. This kind of attitude can be dissected through the concept of resilience as well. According to Tugade and Fredricksson[39], there are individuals who seem to "bounce back" from negative events quite effectively, whereas others are seemingly unable to get out of their negative ruts.

Self-Fulfillment through Action

Knowing what one's signature strengths are is important but not enough. Being able to use these strengths provide the sense of meaningful doing and thus with positive experiences that can at their best lead to the state of flow, the ultimate autotelic experience[see 40]. Therefore, it is also important that people are able to do those things that they can, to fulfill themselves and use their talent, to create and develop. Locke and Latham[41] have called this "high performance cycle": If the challenge includes expectancy of success, high performance is guaranteed assuming that the person is engaged to the goal, receives adequate feedback, and situational factors do not affect the performance considerably[see also 42]. Similar findings have been learned from the various education levels[e.g., 6,43,44] and hobbies[e.g.,45], too.

The Cloudberry Figure of Human Resources and Holistic Positive Development

When the aim is to analyze people's chances to achieve well-being, human resources are one possible way of starting the contemplation. Our understanding is that the above-mentioned four factors form the basis. They can be illustrated as four fundamental human resources in the form of a cloudberry (see Figure 1). Cloudberry is a golden berry of northern swamp areas and a very healthy one. We choose cloudberry for this illustration because as such it already illustrates the outcome of positive development. Its orange and juicy fruit represents the core elements of human resources. The fruit of the cloudberry is at its juiciest when all inner resources have sufficiently developed. Thus, every bit of the cloudberry is considered valuable and important keys to happiness and well-being in life and the healthy development:

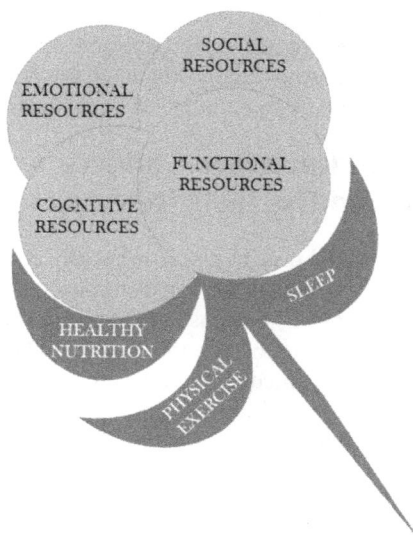

Figure 1. The cloudberry figure of human resources and positive development

(1) Positive feelings enhance intellectual thinking and problem-solving skills, decrease the defending attitude, deliberate, improve memory, and helpfulness. Therefore, they function as emotional resources.

(2) Good interaction skills, empathy, flexibility, patience, caring, and interest are significant social resources that support the creation and preservation of good and close relationships.

(3) Features such as willpower, self-regulation, self-appreciation, and inner motivation are regarded as cognitive resources.

(4) The fourth of the elements is action. At its best, people find joy of doing, sense of meaning, and reach the experiences of flow when they are riveted by tasks where their strengths are employed and where they have the possibility to develop toward the limits of their talents. These kinds of resources are here referred as functional resources.

When a human being is able to get the most of his or her resources, he or she is likely to get positive feedback and recognition from others, succeed, and have increase in his or her self-appreciation. We claim that this kind of positive cycle lays the foundation to healthy development and finding happiness as it represents the true opportunity of self-fulfillment. This positive path is based on the availability of the resources illustrated by the fruit of cloudberry. However, as the illustration (see Figure 1) shows, the fruit does not develop or flourish without proper protection and nurturing. The side leaves of the cloudberry thus manifest the so-called outer elements. Positive and healthy development are threatened without the protective leaves of sleep, nutrition, and physical exercise. They make the use of inner resources possible. And finally, together the fruit and side leaves of a cloudberry make an example of an outcome of beneficial, positive development.

Discussion: How to Enchance Children's and Youngster's Abilities to Find and Use their Resources

Childhood may be the optimal time to promote healthy attitudes, behavior, adjustment, and prevention of problems by, for example, recognizing the children's strengths and building on those strengths[46]. It has been shown that children's development is greatly affected by the phenomena that take place in their growing surroundings: juvenile culture, media, as well as the societal values and ideals. In addition to home[47,48], the surroundings do matter and especially the people being in close contact with children as they influence children's development and growth[e.g., 49,50].

There are various theories of the meaning of positive influence (e.g., encouragement and support) that helps understanding the significance of education atmosphere already in childhood. For example, according to broaden-and-build theory[51], positive emotions, such as joy, interest, contentment, and love, broaden an individual's thought-action repertoire: joy sparks the urge to play, interest sparks the urge to explore, contentment sparks the urge to savor and integrate, and love sparks a recurring cycle of each these urges within safe, close relationships.

According to the post-modern idea of childhood, childhood is a social construction and a child is the constructor of his or her own life, knowledge, identity, and culture[52]. Therefore, development does not happen distinctively in phases nor is it universal as there are cultural variation. At its best, education offers a positive environment that enhances the development of children's strengths that are important to survival in the modern world: Healthy self-confidence and self-esteem, balanced emotional life, judgment and responsibility, the ability to control one's own behavior and make healthy choices, empathy as well as the ability to respect and appreciate other people represent such features[see 53].

Our fast-changing society requires a new kind of professionalism of teachers[54]: the emphasis is on teachers' societal responsibilities and their roles as active future makers[55,56]. According to Coleman[57], good childhood is an important goal of education requiring that more attention is given to children's holistic well-being at school because that lays the foundation of healthy behaviors, healthy choices and lifestyles. We want to end our discussion by quoting Prof. Seligman[15] when he states that flourishing "will be aided by positive education, in which teachers embed the principles of well-being into what they teach, and the depression and anxiety of their students drop and their students' happiness rises"[15, p. 240] and that "when individuals flourish, health, productivity, and peace follow"[15, p. 240]. We as Nordic educators wanted to illustrate the elements of positive development in a form of a cloudberry: healthy and well-balanced, and cherishing the idea of having the resources available for all.

References

1. Haller, M., & Hadler, M. (2006). How social relations and structures can produce happiness and unhappiness: an international comparative analysis. *Social Indicators Research, 75*, 169–216.
2. Webster-Stratton, C., & Reid, M. J. (2004). Strengthening social and emotional competence in young children-the foundation for early school readiness and success: incredible years classroom social skills and problem-solving curriculum. *Infants & Young Children, 17*(2), 96-113.
3. Linley, P. A., Joseph, S., Maltby, J., Harrington, S., & Wood, A. M. (2009). Positive psychology applications. In S. J. Lopez & C. R. Snyder (Eds.), *Oxford handbook of positive psychology* (pp. 35-47). Oxford: Oxford University Press.
4. Schiffrin, H. H., & Nelson, K. Æ S. (2010). Stressed and happy? Investigating the relationship between happiness and perceived stress. *Journal of Happiness Studies, 11*, 33–39.
5. Diener, E., & Seligman, M. E. P. (2004). Beyond money: toward an economy of well-being. *Psychological Science in the Public Interest, 5*(1), 1-31.
6. Gilpin, J. M. (2008). Teaching happiness. The role of positive psychology in the classroom. *Pell Scholars and Senior Theses, 12*, 1-23.

7. Luthans, F., Luthans, K. W., & Luthans, B. C. (2004). Positive psychological capital: Beyond human and social capital. *Business Horizons, 47*(1), 45-50.

8. Luthans, F., Avolio, B. J., Avey, J. B., & Norman, S. M. (2007). Positive psychological capital: Measurement and relationship with performance and satisfaction. *Personnel Psychology, 60*, 541–572.

9. McKee-Ryan, F. M., Song, Z., Wanberg, C. R., & Kinicki, A. J. (2005). Psychological and physical well-being during unemployment: a meta-analytic study. *Journal of Applied Psychology, 90*(1), 53–76.

10. Danziger, S. K., Kalil, A., & Anderson, N. J. (2000). Human capital, physical health, and mental health of welfare recipients: co-occurrence and correlates. *Journal of Social Issues, 56*(4), 635–654.

11. Avey, J. B., Luthans, F., Smith, R. M., & Palmer, N. F. (2010). Impact of positive psychological capital on employee well-being over time. *Journal of Occupational Health Psychology, 15*(1), 17–28.

12. Little, L. M., Simmons, B. L., & Nelson, D. L. (2007). Health among leaders: positive and negative affect, engagement and burnout, forgiveness and revenge. *Journal of Management Studies, 44*(2), 243-260.

13. Edwards, J. R., & Cooper, C. L. (1988). The impacts of positive psychological states on physical health: a review and theoretical framework. *Social Science Medicine, 27*(12), 1147–459.

14. Taylor, S. E., Kemeny, M. E., Reed, G. M., Bower, J. E., & Gruenewald, T. L. (2000). Psychological resources, positive illusions, and health. *American Psychologist, 55*(1), 99-109.

15. Seligman, M. E. P. (2011). *Flourish. A visionary new understanding of happiness and well-being*. New York, NY: Free Press.

16. Diener, E., Suh, E. M., Lucas, R. E., & Smith, H. L. (1999). Subjective well-being: Three decades of progress. *Psychological Bulletin, 125*, 276–302.

17. Diener, E., Lucas, R. E., & Napa Scollon, C. (2006). Beyond the hedonic treadmill. Revising the adaptation theory of well-being. *American Psychologist, 61*(4), 305-314.

18. Magnusson, D., & Mahoney, J. L. (2006). Holistinen lähestymistapa myönteisen kehityksen tutkimuksessa [A holistic perspective on the positive development research]. In L. G. Aspinwall & U. M. Staudinger (Eds.), *Ihmisen vahvuuksien psykologia* [A psychology of human strengths] (pp. 232–250). Helsinki: Edita.

19. Seligman, M. E. P. (2002). *Authentic happiness*. New York, NY: Free Press.

20. Mahoney, M. J. (2002) Constructivism and positive psychology. In C. R. Snyder & S. J. Lopez (Eds.), *Oxford handbook of positive psychology* (pp. 745–750). Oxford: Oxford University Press.

21. Baltes, P. B., & Freund, A. M. (2006). Ihmisen vahvuudet ja viisaus [Human strengths and wisdom]. In L. G. Aspinwall & U. M. Staudinger (Eds.), *Ihmisen vahvuuksien psykologia* [A psychology of human strength] (pp. 34-46). Helsinki: Edita.

22. Pyhältö, K., Soini, T., & Pietarinen, J. (2010). Pupils' pedagogical well-being in comprehensive school—significant positive and negative school experiences of Finnish ninth graders. *European Journal of Psychology of Education, 25*(2), 207-221.

23. Seligman, M. E. P. (2009). Positive education: Positive psychology and classroom interventions. *Oxford Review of Education, 35*(3), 293-311.

24. Huebner, E. S., Gilman, R., Reschly, A. L., & Hall, R. (2009). Positive schools. In S. J. Lopez & C. R. Snyder (Eds.), *Oxford handbook of positive psychology* (pp. 561-568). Oxford: Oxford University Press.

25.   Seligman, M. E. P., Steen, T. A., Park, N., & Peterson, C. (2005). Positive psychology progress. Empirical validation of interventions. *American Psychologist, 60*(5), 410-421.
26.   Seligman, M. E. P., Parks, A. C., & Steen, T. A. (2004). A balanced psychology and a full life. *Philosophical Transactions of the Royal Society B, 359*, 1379–1381.
27.   Määttä, K., & Uusiautti, S. (2012a). The four-leaf clover of human resources. *Research Journal in Organizational Psychology & Educational Studies, 1*(1), 37-42.
28.   Määttä, K., & Uusiautti, S. (2012b). How to learn to enjoy sexuality – the resources of human sexuality. *Advances in Psychology Studies, 1*(1), 8-13.
29.   Isen, A. M., & Reeve, J. (2006). The influence of positive affect on intrinsic and extrinsic motivation: facilitating enjoyment of play, responsible work behavior, and self-control. *Motivation and Emotion, 29*(4), 297 - 325.
30.   Uusiautti, S., & Määttä, K. (2011). The ability to love – a virtue-based approach. *British Journal of Educational Research, 2*(1), 1-19.
31.   Taylor, S. E., & Brown, J. D. (1988). Illusion and well-being: A social psychological perspective on mental health. *Psychological Bulletin, 110*, 193-210.
32.   Seder, J. P., & Oishi, S. (2012). Intensity of smiling in Facebook photos predicts future life satisfaction. *Social Psychological and Personality Science, 3*(4), 407-413.
33.   Kavanagh, D. J., & Bower, G. H. (1985). Mood and self-efficacy: Impact of joy and sadness on perceived capabilities. *Cognitive Therapy and Research, 9*(5), 507-525.
34.   Berscheid, E. (2006). Ihmisen suurin vahvuus: toiset ihmiset [The greatest strength of a human being: other human beings]. In L. G. Aspinwall & U. M. Staudinger (Eds.), *Ihmisen vahvuuksien psykologia* [A psychology of human strengths] (pp. 47–56). Helsinki: Edita.
35.   Rose, R. (2000). How much does social capital add to individual health? A survey study of Russians. *Social Science & Medicine, 51*(9), 1421–1435.
36.   Carver, C. S., & Scheier, M. F. (2002). Optimism. In C. R. Snyder & S. J. Lopez (Eds.), *Oxford handbook of positive psychology* (pp. 231-243). Oxford: Oxford University Press.
37.   Uusiautti, S. (2008). *"Tänään teen elämäni parhaan työn" Työmenestys Vuoden Työntekijöiden kertomana* ["Today, I'll work better than ever" Success at work described by the employees of the year]. (PhD Diss, University of Lapland, Rovaniemi, Finland.)
38.   Uusiautti, S., & Määttä, K. (2011). Love for work as the way towards well-being. *Global Journal of Human Social Science, 11*(9), 63-68.
39.   Tugade, M. M., & Fredricksson, B. L. (2004). Resilient individuals use positive emotions to bounce back from negative emotional experiences. *Journal of Personality and Social Psychology, 86*(2), 320–333.
40.   Csikszentmihalyi, M. (2008). *Flow. The psychology of optimal experience.* (10th ed.) New York, NY: HarperPerennial.
41.   Locke, E. A., & Latham, G. P. (1990). Work motivation and satisfaction: light at the end of the tunnel. *Psychological Science, 1*(4), 240-246.
42. Uusiautti, S. (2013). On the positive connection between success and happiness. *International Journal of Research Studies in Psychology, 3*(1), 1-11.
43.   Green, J., Liem G. A., Martin, A. J., Colmar, S., Marsh, H. W., & McInerney, D. (2012). Academic motivation, self-concept, engagement and performance in high school: Key processes from a longitudinal perspective. *Journal of Adolescence, 35*(5), 1111-1122.
44.   Oades, L. G., Robinson, P., Green, S., & Spence, G. B. (2011). Towards a positive university. *The Journal of Positive Psychology, 6*(6), 432-439.
45.   Carruthers, C., & Hood, C. D. (2005). The power of positive psychology. *Parks & Recreation, Oct 2005*, 30-37.
46.   Brown Kirschman, K. J., Johnson, R. J., Bender, J. A., & Roberts, M. C. (2009). Positive psychology for children and adolescents: Development, prevention, and promotion. In S. J.

140

Lopez & C. R. Snyder (Eds.), *Oxford handbook of positive psychology* (pp. 133–147). Oxford, NY: Oxford University Press.

47.   Kyrönlampi-Kylmänen, T., & Määttä K. (2011a). What do the children really think about a day-care centre – The 5 to 7-years-old Finnish children speak out. *Early Child Development and Care, 182*(5), 505-520.

48.   Kyrönlampi-Kylmänen, T., & Määttä K. (2011b). What is it like to be at home – The experiences of 5 to 7-year old Finnish children. *Early Child Development and Care, 182*(1), 71-86.

49.   Hagegull, B., & Bohlin, G. (1995). Day care quality, family and child characteristics and socioemotional development. *Early Childhood Research Quarterly, 10*, 505–526.

50.   Boshcee, M. A., & Jacobs, G. (1997). *Ingredients for quality child care.* National Network for Child Care.
http://www.nncc.org/choose.quality.care/ingredients.html#anchor143569

51.   Fredrickson, B. L. (2004). The broaden-and-build theory of positive emotions. *Philosophical Transactions of the Royal Society B, 359*, 1367–1377.

52.   Kronqvist, E.-L., & Kumpulainen, K. (2011). *Lapsuuden oppimisympäristöt. Eheä polku varhaiskasvatuksesta kouluun* [Childhood learning environments. Harmonious path from early education to school]. Helsinki: WSOYpro.

53.   Määttä, K. (2007). Vanhempainrakkaus – suurin kaikista [Parental love –the greatest love]. In K. Määttä (Ed.), *Helposti särkyvää. Nuoren kasvun turvaaminen* [Fragile – Securing youngsters' growth] (pp. 220–236). Helsinki: Kirjapaja.

54.   Paksuniemi, M., Uusiautti, S., & Määttä, K. (2013). *What are Finnish teachers made of? A glance at teacher education in Finland yesterday and today.* New York, NY: Nova Science Publishers.

55.   von Wright, M. (2009). The shunned essentials of pedagogy: Authority, love and mystery. *Nordic Philosophy of Education Network NERA Annual Meeting*, Trondheim, March 5-7th 2009. http://oru.diva-portal.org/smash/record.jsf?pid=diva2:212954

56.   Seidl, B., & Friend, G. (2002). Leaving authority at the door: Equal-status community-based experiences and the preparation of teachers for diverse classrooms. *Teaching and Teacher Education, 18*, 421-433.

57.   Coleman, J. (2009). Well-being in schools: Empirical measure, or politician's dream? *Oxford Review of Education, 35*(3), 281–292.

www.ingramcontent.com/pod-product-compliance
Lightning Source LLC
Chambersburg PA
CBHW031541260326
41914CB00002B/218